TRAGER
for Self-Healing

TRAGER
for Self-Healing

A Practical Guide
for Living in the Present Moment

AUDREY MAIRI

Foreword by Deane Juhan, author of *Job's Body*

H J KRAMER

published in a joint venture with

NEW WORLD LIBRARY
NOVATO, CALIFORNIA

An H J Kramer Book
published in a joint venture with
New World Library

Editorial office:
P.O. Box 1082
Tiburon, California 94920

Administrative office:
14 Pamaron Way
Novato, California 94949

Edited by Nancy Grimley Carleton, Candis Graham, and Paul Latour
Text design and typography by Tona Pearce Myers

Library of Congress Cataloging-in-Publication Data
Mairi, Audrey
Trager for self-healing : a practical guide for living in the present moment / Audrey Mairi. — 1st ed.
    p. cm.
Includes bibliographical references and index.
ISBN-13: 978-1-932073-19-5 (pbk. : alk. paper)
1. Exercise. 2. Mind and body. I. Title.
RA781.M337 2006
613—dc22   2006017637

First printing, September 2006
ISBN-10: 1-932073-19-1
ISBN-13: 978-1-932073-19-5
Printed in Canada on acid-free, partially recycled paper.

Distributed by Publishers Group West

10   9   8   7   6   5   4   3   2   1

This book is lovingly dedicated to my two mentors:

My Trager mentor,
Karen Hortig,
September 7, 1945–May 10, 2005

My writing mentor,
Candis Graham,
February 14, 1949–November 22, 2005

There is a way of being
Which is lighter
Which is freer
A way in which work
As well as play
Becomes a dance
And living a song
We can learn this way

— MILTON TRAGER

CONTENTS

MENTASTICS (MENTAL GYMNASTICS)

FOREWORD

*It is natural for the mind to move
towards the fields of greater happiness.*

— MAHARISHI MAHESH YOGI

I f the above statement is true, then pressing questions immediately arise: Why are our minds — and through them our bodies — so obviously susceptible to unhappiness, inner conflicts, unnecessarily contentious relations with others, fear, pain, chronic conditions, degenerative disorders, and the rest of the host of demons that plague us? What so distances us from our natural heritage, handed down to us through millennia of evolutionary development, of keen self-awareness, effective self-regulation, and successful adaptation? What are the obstacles that divert us from the joys of learning, from an enthusiastic curiosity about ourselves, from a more conscious engagement with our past, our present, and the possibilities of our future? What are the pitfalls that trap us and disable the powerful resources of self-healing that nature has given us?

Here is a book that directly addresses these questions and offers important answers drawn from the author's twenty-something years of practical experience in self-healing, bodywork, counseling, and teaching. And more important, here are a book and a depth of insight that offer simple principles and practical steps to follow on your personal journey out of those negative susceptibilities and around those obstacles and pitfalls. What you have in your hands is a map toward the rediscovery of the powerful resources within every one of us, resources that have been hamstrung by the intense stress from the industrialization and technologizing of our lives, and by the educational, medical, and spiritual models that have been given to us. Through mutual reinforcement and self-fulfilling prophesy, these models have become the core of our acculturated beliefs about our minds, our bodies, and our capacities for self-healing. Their underlying and debilitating message is that effective alternatives are not possible and that other than seeking expert intervention, there is little to nil that we can do to better our lot. What Audrey Mairi tells us is that this just ain't so.

In his novel *Jitterbug Perfume*, Tom Robbins writes that as a guide to regulating human behavior, the Ten Commandments are redundant; we really need only one: "Lighten up." In the midst of the multitasking demands on our modern lives and the consequent self-expectations we levy against ourselves, we have lost sight of the potentials for self-development and healing. These are not resources that can be forced upon us or made to emerge under pressure. The hurly-burly social forces around us and the emotional pressures within us are the very things that have obscured them. It is useless to strive for them the way we have learned to strive for everything else in our lives. Instead, we must slow down. We must pause. We must listen to ourselves. We must cultivate an inner quiet wherein the unconscious wisdom of our bodies can reemerge more consciously in our lives.

The work developed and passed on by Dr. Milton Trager was the result of a lifetime of learning to cultivate this slowing down, this pausing, this quiet questioning of the body and active engagement with the answers it offers. Audrey Mairi has been a longtime student and practitioner of Dr. Trager's work, and it — along with her successful resolutions while on her own personal journey of healing and teaching — deeply informs what she has to say here. The work is not a technique, a protocol, a procedure, a formula, or an intervention. It is a learning: learning to slow down, to pause, and to find that inner quiet from which the answers to our pains and dilemmas can emerge from the natural wisdom — the impulse toward greater happiness — that is our heritage.

Audrey Mairi's book is the most thorough and accurate description of the Trager Approach that I have ever read. The successful use of this book will require active engagement on the part of the reader. It will be to no avail if you simply read it, close it, and say, "I got it." Let your reading be an opening to a doing, to a practice and refinement of the simple but powerfully effective meditations in awareness and movement you will find here. And why not? The engagement called for here is with yourself — the most accessible and most important person in your life. So take this book home not as a weekend read but as a long-term companion. As they say in Alcoholics Anonymous, "Keep coming back; it works if you work it." Here is a guide out of the cul-de-sac of impotence and debilitation. Work it. Lighten up.

Deane Juhan,
Senior Trager instructor and author of
Job's Body and *Touched by the Goddess*

Taking Flight

We all have feelings of fear and doubt, even authors of self-help books, but by *showing up* and *being present* these supposedly "negative" feelings can lead to small decisions that, in turn, manifest a new lightness of being. To illustrate, let me tell you the story of how this book first took flight. This story will reveal how it is possible to change overwhelming, painful situations into blissful moments of wonder that show us we *can* choose differently!

Like many stories, this one starts with the protagonist, me, feeling overwhelmed, lost, alone, and in pain. Like the inside of a golf ball, I was twisted and jumbled and tight, behaving like the victim I thought I was. My twenty-year marriage had just failed, my dearest friend had unceremoniously dumped me, I had a constant lower backache, my old symptoms of shingles had flared up, my stomach was in knots, and I seemed to have lost the knowledge and ability to make empowered decisions. I was brokenhearted and at a crossroads: I could give in to victimhood, or I could invite in the healing light.

This choice was clearly presented to me during a phone call from a dear friend and colleague in Easton, Pennsylvania. "Come visit," she said. "Why not?"

"Because I can't afford it," I replied. "I just returned from visiting my family on the other side of the country, and I can't spend more money jetting off again for no other reason than to visit a friend."

"Aren't you worth it?" she asked.

"Yes, but I'm feeling so pressured and afraid," I confessed. "How can I justify spending more money when I don't know if I can support myself?"

"But I'll buy your ticket."

This statement left me with a jumble of emotions: gratitude for being "rescued," humility and embarrassment at the possibility of accepting her help and exposing my vulnerability, plus a distinct residue of fear.

"Well... I'll think about it," I replied.

"Don't forget to breathe," my friend said. "Stay present and you'll find your way."

My chest rose and fell with her suggestion. "Thank you for the reminder," I affirmed. "I *will* think about it."

After I hung up, it was decision time. I paused. I wanted to heal. But I had a problem. I didn't know how. I had no answers. I didn't even have questions! It was clear I wasn't going to *figure* my way out of this one. So what could I do? I decided I would listen to my friend and combine mindful awareness with physical sensations. I would become aware of the Life Force. To the best of my ability, I would not muddy it with expectations of the future or judgments about the past. I would use some of the underlying principles of the Trager Approach to body/mind integration.

I decided to release the weight of my troubles — if only for a moment — and focus on my body. Standing in my living room in Ottawa, I noticed the bottoms of my feet on the plush carpet. I felt my rib cage open and close with each breath. I shifted my weight gently back and forth and then from side to side, finding my center of gravity. I imagined a string attached to the top of my head, tenderly lifting my bones skyward. Then I fancied myself with a long dinosaur tail that gave me tripodlike stability.

I asked myself, *What could be lighter?*

Miraculously, within seconds a sensation of lightness flooded through me. With it were no answers, no revelations, only a feeling of peace — the power of the Life Force.

A few days later my friend's persuasive voice came across the wires again. "I've talked to my travel agent and there's a seat sale," she said.

Just the sound of her voice caused me to recall the pleasurable, peaceful sensation I had experienced after our last conversation. I took a deep breath that went right to my toes and with my out-breath felt as if I were rising like a balloon. I experienced the peace and clarity of the Life Force and in a heartbeat knew that this was a wonderful opportunity.

I won't give in to my fears, I announced to myself. "Yes, I'll do it!" I announced to my friend.

Without *thinking*, I simply chose what felt right. Although I had no idea of it at the time, this decision would affect the direction of my life.

Three weeks later the day of my flight arrived, and I embarked upon the short journey to Pennsylvania, excited that soon I would see someone I loved and felt safe with. While flying I gave myself permission to *not know* what was going to happen. I was a beginner, starting over with a clean slate.

Stepping off the plane onto the tarmac, I turned my face to the sun, closed my eyes, and took a deep breath. The area behind my eyelids felt warm. The soft air in my nostrils still smelled like summer, gently erasing the hint of fall I had left behind in Ottawa. After my friend welcomed me affectionately, we traveled to the picturesque town of Easton and her fabulous Frank Lloyd Wright home, where I settled into the upstairs guest room.

As I finished unpacking, I realized I was building an agenda about what I needed to do and say. I reminded myself to let go of my expectations about this visit. *I only need to be a beginner*, I told myself as I made my way downstairs. *I can start fresh; I don't have to hold on to the past*, I repeated as I went out the front door. *I don't have to have all the answers*, I reassured myself as I meandered through my friend's heavily wooded suburban neighborhood. *I just need to be here now.*

Instead of pressuring myself, I simply noticed my feet pacing the earth. I felt the weight of my arms swinging at my sides and the rhythmic movement of my gait. Soon I felt a profound bond with the charming and uniquely styled homes surrounded by manicured lawns and lush gardens. One house in particular caught my attention, and I stopped to look at it more closely. It was a sprawling, two-story home perched upon a small hill. On both its front corners stone turrets stood sentinel, while throughout the rest of the structure an eclectic mixture of arched, round, and rectangular mullioned windows added a sense of magic. The wooden siding was a mellow shade of yellow, while a darker tone of the same color trimmed the doors, windows, and wrap-around porch.

A large calico cat, sensing my presence, lazily raised her head from her sleeping position on the porch to peer at me. Figuring that I was probably harmless, she decided to get a closer look. She gracefully rose, stretched, and padded down the front steps, rambled over the curving walkway, and stood under the pale peach-tipped roses that covered the arbor at the entrance to this incredible house. Satisfied that I was indeed no threat, she pivoted in an act of dismissal and strolled into the garden. I watched her as she passed clusters of fiery red, burnt orange, and buttery yellow late-blooming flowers and settled in the shade under the sprawling ferns. Just then the scent of soothing lavender rode on the breath of the sudden breeze.

I inhaled deeply. I was connected.

Such a beautiful place; a child could have a field day here, I thought while lingering at the edge of the property. Then I imagined myself as a young girl trapped in one of the stone turrets waiting desperately for a knight in shining armor to gallop down the path, white horse and all, to rescue me. While smiling at this childhood daydream, it occurred to me that this was exactly how I had felt back in Ottawa — a damsel in distress trapped in a tower of grief — and it was this feeling that had brought me to Pennsylvania. To think that I almost hadn't come, hadn't listened to my friend — my female knight in shining armor — who suggested I *Hook-Up* to the light (to use the Trager term for connecting to the Life

Force). She knew this would help me realize how important it was to take this time for myself.

She was right, of course. I needed a breather from the trauma of my recent divorce and all the explanations to family and friends that went with it. I needed a way to bring perspective back into my life. I mentally patted myself on the back for taking these few minutes to feel the Life Force flowing through me.

With a lighter, freer step I returned from exploring my friend's neighborhood and brewed myself a cup of tea. Then, just as I was about to sit down in the glassed-in sunroom, my breath caught in my throat. There, by the woods at the edge of the property, standing proudly on the shady succulent grass, was a stag. His compelling presence drew me out onto the patio, where I gently placed my cup on the table and quietly sat on a wrought-iron chair. Staying as still as I could, barely breathing, I was eventually rewarded by the sight of a doe and her children coming to join "Poppa."

Rich woodland smells saturated my nostrils and birdsong filled my ears. I closed my eyes and felt the heat of the sun dance behind my lids and along my skin. A long, cleansing sigh escaped my lips. I felt connected to my environment, at one with the trees, the grass, the birds, the deer. I was linked to the Life Force in such a profound way I couldn't even feel the seat of the chair as being separate from my bottom. I sank deeper and deeper into myself, then freely, lightly, playfully looked inside. *How still my inner world feels compared to the turmoil of my outer world back in Ottawa. This woodland setting is so perfect — tranquil yet vibrating with life. Definitely food for my grieving soul. Sure wouldn't take much to get some creativity flowing here.*

My next thought came out of nowhere: *I think I'll write a book.*

My eyelids flew open and I sat up straight. *A book? Why, I've never written anything substantial in my life — just a handful of poems done years ago and bits and pieces for my weekly writing group. Would that qualify as enough experience to write a book?* My fears surfaced immediately. *What on earth would I write about? What makes me think I can write something so enormous? Who wants to hear what I have to say? What do I have to say?* The doubts came fast and furious, but before my fears got the better of me, I remembered to pause... and trust....

I took a deep breath....

I wiggled my toes....

I felt the Life Force....

I let go of my fears... and snuggled deeper into the chair.

I indulged my musings.

Immediately my friend popped into my mind, which brought my thoughts to our mutual love of Trager. I reflected on my Trager practice and how I chose this profession because of its holistic approach to wellness. But because this approach is hard to define to the general public, the Trager organization seemed to me to be leaning toward the medical explanation of our work, allowing the energetic mechanics to fade gently into the background.

It was then I realized: I wanted more. I wanted to dive even deeper. I wanted to explore Trager's spiritual potential. I wanted to know what enlightenment felt like in my body.

My thoughts raced. Ideas tripped over themselves in a rush to become conscious.

I know this subject, I thought. *I've eaten and slept Trager for over twenty years. I've inhaled it and exhaled it. I've fought it, I've been bored with it, I've taught it, and I've incorporated it into my everyday life. I can use myself as an example. I can take my readers on a journey. Give them Trager tools to rediscover their body/mind. Help them feel connected to the light that sustains us all. I can inspire readers to change from identifying with fear and a sense of being overwhelmed and victimized, to empowerment and magical moments of wonder. Yes, I can do this! I can write a book!*

As I sat on the patio a smile formed slowly around my eyes, worked its way about my head, kissed my lips, then spiraled dizzily inside my body. I felt tingly, clear, energized, saturated with light.

My mind raved on in excitement: *Using the Trager Approach requires very little of our precious time, no religious conversion, no dramatic changes in diet, no gadgets to plug in, no psychic abilities, no strenuous training program. It works as well for the young as for the aged, for the couch potato as for the athlete. But it is more than even that. It provides a safe environment to gently and painlessly "melt" areas of physical and emotional inflexibility. It uses fundamentally simple principles as tools to connect to the Life Force in a conscious way. And this paves the way for spiritual awareness.*

So many paths to self-awareness ask us to ignore, detach from, or rise above the physical body. But Trager is a holistic approach because it incorporates our body into the spiritual package. To do this, we meet the Life Force where it resides, in the present moment, our point of power. Trager forges this last conscious link to our source. It is, my inner dialogue concluded, *quite simply, the perfect blueprint for living gracefully in an enlightened state in the physical body.*

I liked the sound of that so much I said it out loud: "The Trager Approach is the perfect blueprint for living gracefully in an enlightened state in the physical body."

At that moment on that patio, I knew I could — no, I knew I needed to — do this. The Trager Approach has been a gift in my life, a gift that welcomed back the awareness of the Life Force into my body and therefore into my waking experience. I wanted to share this gift because the more I share the awareness of the Life Force, the more it grows within me. All doubts erased, I rushed to grab my favorite pen and notebook.

And I wrote:

I am a living work of art
An organic creation of light
The organ of consciousness.

A conduit for sound
Music flows through me
Creating movement and expression.

Through my sight
Form and color manifest
In natural landscapes.

Aroma settles in my cells
Stirring memories
Scent: an interpreter of my past.

The earth and my body
Synergistically linked
Together we are One.

Through feeling the light
I anchor the experience
Of the physical to the Divine.

I am a living work of art
In the process of becoming
Consciously united with All.

Playing Light

Early morning sunlight streams through a giant stained-glass window. The warm bitter aroma of coffee rises from take-out paper cups. Mouths gape in tired yawns. Knuckles rub against eye sockets.

"Everyone! Take your places please."

Three hundred people amble onto the stage — basses to one side, tenors to the other, and, opposite us altos, the sopranos. We are the Victoria Gettin' Higher Choir, rehearsing for our winter concert to support the Earth Charter and the Power of Hope youth program.

We begin with an in-breath, breathing into our feet, calling up the energy from the earth to nourish and ground us. Riding the tone of the out-breath is all the fatigue and stress that has found harbor in our body. We do it again: sound vibration hunting out the last traces of restriction in bellies and chests. Our arms rise on the in-breath, drawing in finer, subtler energies; our crown chakras open to all the light filtering through the rainbow-colored mandala set in the immense window before us. We let our arms float down, leaving our chests open and free. We are using our bodies to sing, not just our voices. Each focused movement asks, *How open can my voice become? How freely can my body express this?*

We rehearse the entire first half of the concert, getting the timing just right, working hard with the children's choir from Kid Power. Their high, clear voices send shivers down my spine. Both choirs blend and harmonize, sending out a heartfelt plea through song to save the planet. Later, during a break, I sit in the front pew, full from singing — feeling soft, open, energized.

Our guest performer for this concert will be Raffi. Though I have yet to see him, I know of him. Raffi is the children's troubadour who spawned the "Baby Beluga" generation in Canada. So when a sweet-smiling, soulful-eyed stranger sporting a salt-and-pepper beard beneath dark, close-cropped hair bounds like a gazelle onto the stage, I assume it must be Raffi. He pauses, looks around, and says, "Hi! Thank you for letting me be part of this."

We all beam as if it were our decision alone to have him with us onstage at this winter concert. He walks up to the mike and starts to sing in a clear voice: "In this world of wonder, circle where we all belong — can I have more mike on the guitar?" he asks, after which the soundman and he play back and forth until Raffi is satisfied. Once again, he begins to warm up.

I listen with half a mind. The other half I let roam until something catches my attention. It is not his timely, aware, profound lyrics. It is not the sound of his warm, inviting open voice. It is not even the creative, stirring, upbeat musical score. What I am attracted to is his movement — soft and fluffy, almost ethereal. He is ever so lightly bouncing on the balls of his feet, shifting his weight from one side to the other, becoming lighter and lighter, like a bubble bouncing along an updraft. He oozes lightness from every pore — I think surely he will drift away.

The radiant feeling is catchy, and I get it — an *ah ha!* Yes, *that* feeling — thank you. Like a river it flows deeply into my chest and belly, wending its way to my feet, spreading into my toes. I feel spacious, buoyant, playful — joyous! This new layer of experience washes upon my senses like fresh spring rain upon my upturned face. Effortlessly I have caught the gift of lightness from Raffi.

※

This feeling stayed with me throughout the rest of the rehearsal. I easily recalled it when I was inspired to sit at my computer to write the introduction to this book. Settling into my chair in front of the monitor, I closed my eyes, breathed in deeply, and asked myself, *How did I feel watching Raffi this morning?* Almost instantly my upper chest lightened, my back lengthened, and I sat up straighter but . . . easier. A smile of contentment played around my mouth. I paused, my hands hovering over the keys.

What is light?

I was intrigued.

You strike a match or flick a switch and — *presto* — darkness is gone. In our inner world light brings clarity, comfort, peace. When light is blocked in the outer world, we experience cold shadows, lack of color, impaired vision. When it is impeded in our inner world, we become frustrated, confused, and unstable.

We also recognize light as a particular physical sensation. What does it feel like? Hold a bag of flour; then hold a feather. Observe a gossamer-winged butterfly perched on a flower petal, and take into your body the answer to *What is light?* Listen to the song of a harp. Notice how some people appear to float rather than walk — as if they have springs in their feet that enable them to play with gravity rather than be weighed down by it.

Raffi was such a person. He didn't have to do anything except be present in *himself,* just as I didn't have to do anything to receive it but be present in *myself.* The founder of Trager Psychophysical Integration, Dr. Milton Trager, used to say that you catch the feeling of lightness, ease, and presence from someone who already has it. It's like catching the measles. And I have found this to be true.

About This Book

I have been a seeker of self-awareness my whole life. I realized early on that with awareness comes a lightness of being, and with this light comes healing and peace. Over the years I have found some very simple, practical ways to carry my light with me wherever I go and into whatever situation I find myself. These simple practices are based on the underlying principles of the Trager Approach; they work not only for Trager practitioners but also for all of us who seek more lightness in our life.

I wrote *Trager for Self-Healing* to share these concepts with you. I hope you will find that they demythologize enlightenment — taking it out of the realm of the religious or supernatural and into the everyday world without a lot of fancy medical, intellectual, or spiritual jargon. I've structured the book in three parts. Part 1: The Basics, gives a foundation of knowledge, leading you through a series of concepts and stories that will help you understand how the Trager Approach to body/mind and Spirit integration works, and why it is so effective. In Part 2: Tools to Get There, we get physical. Here I teach six simple yet powerful tools that will help you consciously feel the Life Force flowing through your body, fostering a state of presence. Part 3: Putting It All Together, consists of real-life stories that put these concepts into practice, illustrating the practical and versatile nature of the Trager Approach. The interludes between the parts simply provide a chance to pause and reflect on what we've covered so far and point toward what comes next.

It is your birthright to feel good about who you are and what you are meant to do while in your body. You *can* have a feeling of peace, even if you have responsibilities and are overworked — stretched to the limit. Think about it! Wouldn't it be wonderful to be released from bad thoughts, problem people, and difficult situations? Wouldn't it be grand to connect, in an instant, to that parting of the clouds we all crave when we are bogged down?

This book will help remind you how to connect with the light; it will give entry to your personal sunbeam. You will gain access to the source of lightness — the creative force behind everything you do. I don't mean that all of a sudden you will go out and buy oil paints and brushes. I mean that part-nered with your body/mind is a creative energetic force that effortlessly assists in the orchestration of your everyday life. When consciously invited into your body/mind, this creative energy brings lightness, joy, good health, and, most of all, peace.

Trager for Self-Healing offers a door, an access portal to the present moment. Being present is not an intellectual process; it is a sensation, an experience. Once we know *how*, we can recall it again and again.

This book can be your guide when life becomes too much. You will learn how to access the Life Force and anchor the state of *presence*. You will learn how to easily recall

- what lighter, clearer, and freer *feels* like;
- what being stable in a time of crisis *feels* like;
- what making a healthy choice *feels* like;
- what empowerment *feels* like.

Step into the present, and invite the light into your world. Help bring peace to the planet, one person at a time. Are you ready to shine?

PART ONE

THE BASICS

Not until we experience it
Is it more than just words.

After we experience it
There is no need for words.

The value of words
Is to stimulate
The desire to experience.

— MILTON TRAGER

CHAPTER ONE

So, What *Is* Trager Anyway?

The Trager Approach uses touch and physical movement to invite the body/mind to experience feelings of lightness, of softness, of bliss through something called *Hook-Up*. "Hook-Up is a state of being," Dr. Milton Trager said on many occasions. "It is a Hook-Up of this power that you are surrounded by. It is a life-giving, life-regulating power that has always been there and will always be there. And you can't try to get it. You can't try to Hook-Up because to try is to fail. You don't try. To try is effort, and effort is tension. We don't try. We just allow it to happen. You are going to feel. It is not the moves I do or the technique. Drop the word *technique*. [Trager] is not a technique. It is something different."[1]

This quotation captures the core of the Trager Approach. Yes, there are many "moves" and "techniques" a Trager practitioner learns — the training is intensive — but they are merely the craft of our trade. Just as a writer knows grammar and a guitarist knows chords, a Trager practitioner knows the body — its muscles, bones, and tissue. Such knowledge, however, is not enough, just as knowing grammar or chords is not enough to make great literature or toe-tapping music. To turn craft into something different, something more, something that transcends our limited understanding, a Trager practitioner needs to be able to Hook-Up to the life-giving, life-regulating power that is everywhere at all times. It is for this reason that Dr. Trager suggested we "drop the word *technique*." Dr. Trager knew that at a certain point his students had to let go of their training, stay out of their own way, and get into Hook-Up by arriving in the present moment. In a state of presence, feelings of lightness, softness, and bliss infuse the body/mind, turning technique into an effortless vehicle to transfer these feelings into the client's body and therefore mind.

This is why the Trager Approach (also known as Trager Psychophysical Integration) operates through pleasurable, effortless, easy movement, which softly and safely introduces the body/mind to what it would be like if it were free to function without restriction.

Dr. Milton Trager's Story

When Dr. Trager was young he developed his muscles and sharpened his movement as an amateur acrobat, performing stunts with his brother on the beaches of Miami. But while his brother asked the question "Who can jump the highest?" Milton asked, "Who can land the softest?"

As a result of this way of thinking, he became fascinated with the light, dancelike movements of boxers, and at the age of eighteen he started training under a man named Mickey

Martin. One fateful day Mickey looked like he needed to receive a rubdown rather than give one.

"Lie down, Mickey," young Milton said. "Let me take care of you for a change." A complete novice at bodywork, Milton let his hands innocently explore.

"Where did you learn to do that?" an amazed Mickey asked afterward.

"Well, you taught me."

"I never taught you anything like that, kid, but I don't care. Let me tell you, you got hands!"

Intrigued by this newfound talent, Milton practiced on his family and neighbors. His first patient was his father, who had been suffering from sciatica for two years. After Milton "worked" on him for two weeks, he never had symptoms of sciatica again.

✤

Was it his technique that made such a dramatic difference to his father's health? At this stage in Milton's development, undoubtedly not. It was his ability to Hook-Up while in the present moment, an ability we all have. In fact, it is our birthright, our natural way of being. Unfortunately, as we age many of us forget what this life-regulating power from our source feels like. It falls into the background, soon becoming hindered by ego-based beliefs, then all but forgotten. Most of us shake our heads in wonder when asked what it feels like in our body to be connected with our source.

One way to get a direct experience of this feeling is to engage in a wholehearted application of the exercises provided in this book. Another way is to catch it (like catching the measles, to use the metaphor offered earlier, except without the fever, itch, and skin eruptions) from someone who has got it. A Trager practitioner is just such a person.

A Trager Session

If you were to have a Trager session, you would find that no oils or lotions are used. You would lie passively on a well-padded table (clothed or partially unclothed) while the practitioner, who is consciously Hooked-Up, gently rocks, compresses, elongates, jiggles, and shimmers the tissue in your body. You would experience the practitioner playing along the border of restriction and freedom, inviting into your tissue feelings of lightness, of softness, of bliss.

The session would soon become a movement reeducation that addressed the physical and nonphysical aspects of your body/mind, thereby giving you (whether you knew it or not) an alternative to any erroneous physical and mental patterns you might be holding onto. Through the deep but nonintrusive touch that is Trager's signature, your practitioner would introduce you to the place of all possibility, to the *origin* of everything you have ever thought, felt, or imagined, to that life-giving, life-regulating power all around us. You would know this by the expansive open feeling in your tissue, as if the gravity holding you down had lessened. You would know this by how your joints would seem to have been lubricated, how your breath would deepen, how your mind would quiet. The combination of the practitioner's skill at the craft plus their ability to stand in the present moment (and thereby Hook-Up to source) allows for such a transference.

Dr. Trager taught his students how to stand effortlessly in presence — the state of mind that gives the Trager Approach its magic and power. He developed ways for *anyone* to put him- or herself quickly and effortlessly in the present moment, automatically eliciting the feeling of Hook-Up. He called these tools *Mentastics* (a term coined by his wife, Emily, from the words *mental gymnastics*).

In Dr. Trager's opinion, it is just as important — if not more important — to use Mentastics after the session, off the table (or if you're unable to get a session) to allow the learning process in the nervous system to continue. Mentastics take very little time and are performed alongside everything else we do. In fact, when we use Mentastics throughout our day — washing dishes, making phone calls, walking to the mall — we not only regain and reinforce the feelings received during a session, we also independently foster our growth into presence. The more we stand in presence, the more the feeling of connection to our source grows, the more we are fed this energy, the clearer our decisions, the more relaxed and the healthier our body, the more creative our mind. Each of us can experience these lingering effects of the Trager Approach to body/mind integration by repeatedly practicing the Mentastics presented in this book.

CHAPTER TWO

Giving Yourself Permission to Be a Beginner

It's a competitive world out there," I've heard people say. "Where am I in relation to the next person? Is he ahead of me or behind me? Is she going faster or slower? Does he have more flair, greater interpersonal skills, superior networking abilities? Will she usurp my position? If I don't come up to speed, I'll fall behind. I must do better."

What pressure!

Most people, including me, experience such thoughts, adhering to the belief, either consciously or unconsciously, that we have to perform perfectly immediately upon being given a new task. It is not a great leap to see how our minds become preoccupied, our energy undermined, and our perception narrowed the more we are burdened by comparisons, past mistakes, and future expectations. Such burdens build walls that box in our beliefs and confine our cognitive skills. In turn our creativity and decision-making abilities are hampered.

All of this starts with our upbringing, with the ways we learn to understand the world around us. When I was a child, the only praise and recognition I remember getting came when I got high marks in school. I interpreted this to mean that when I did exceptionally well, I would be recognized and loved (a good thing). When I didn't do well, my young mind reasoned, I would be a failure and not loved (a bad thing).

By adulthood the extensions of this dysfunctional logic had turned me into a perfectionist. I expected myself to perform the first time around — perfectly. Such dogged determination inevitably spilled over to other areas of my life: I tried too hard to learn, tried too hard to relax, to work, to play. I was exhausted all the time!

After a couple of decades of this I started to wonder if there was a more efficient way of being. A better state of mind, maybe? A way to do less and accomplish more?

I found there was. Trager calls it *Beginner's Mind*.

With Beginner's Mind, we approach everything with innocence, loosening expectations based on past experiences and looking at life as if it were fresh and brand-new. This attitude takes us out of the pressure cooker and washes away self-doubt. We become more attentive and more relaxed when we give ourselves permission to *not* know, *not* expect, *not* compare. We no longer prematurely slam the gates on all the information it is possible to gather at any one time. Suddenly, we take in more of what people are communicating. We notice not only their words but also their tonality and their body language: Is that a quiver beneath his bravado? Do those raised shoulders and that sunken chin match the courageous words we're hearing?

It is easy to allow our preconceived notions to cloud our judgments and take us out of what *is*. Such was my experience during my first Trager training.

※

It was a hot, muggy week in July 1984. I was shy and scared. For the first time in eight years I was out in the world by myself. I'd spoken to virtually no one except my second husband and my five- and seven-year-old sons for so long that I couldn't look anyone in the eye. Glancing at the other participants in the church basement, I saw laughter and confidence. Staring down at my old and tattered clothing, I saw inadequacy. We were so poor I had to borrow the money to pay for the course, so I *had* to be good at it! I *had* to be able to justify the disruption I had caused in everyone's life when I chose to do this.

Three days into the course, the class was practicing new ways to move the chest and belly. "Okay," our instructor informed us, "your lower hand fits quite nicely on these lower ribs. Notice how your middle finger points toward the navel. Now, your upper hand is the one that is going to be traveling a bit. First of all, fit the palm of your upper hand on the ball of the shoulder with your fingers pointing in toward the heart. Now, with the movement starting from your feet, rock your pelvis. Then, keeping the upper hand on the ball of the shoulder, point your fingers down the arm and continue to rock the body."

I thought I was doing exactly what she said to do. My hands were in the right position. But my partner wasn't moving! I wasn't getting it. My frustration level, like a kettle about to boil over, bubbled and bubbled until I exploded into tears of defeat and humiliation. My partner thought I was crying because of something she said or did and so was almost brought to tears herself.

The instructor came over and sandwiched my solar plexus between her hands and let me cry. "I don't know how to do this," I wailed. "I'm never going to get it! It's hopeless!" Utterly embarrassed, I continued to sob in front of all those people I barely knew. I wanted to be able to place my hands just so, to move my partner's body this way and that, and — voilà! — have a miracle performed right before my eyes (and everyone else's). I wanted everyone to marvel at my specialness. I wanted to be perfect.

After my tears were spent, the instructor led me in a few Mentastics. She had me feel the bottoms of my feet, sit on my imaginary tail, and think of my torso as an umbrella. With each in-breath I was to open the umbrella, then close it with each out-breath. She quietly told me, "It's okay not to be an expert right off the bat. Not grasping something on the first attempt doesn't mean you're slow or in any way inadequate. It's merely an indicator for you to open up to the moment, release past expectations, and accept that your unique learning style needs space and time to grow."

"Unique learning style?"

"Each of us has her own way of taking in information," she said. "Each of us has her own timing for processing it. Personally I learn by doing. I have to get the feel of something in my *guts* to really know it. Seeing it demonstrated helps, so does hearing the instructions and understanding the reasons behind it, but nothing falls into place for me until I've processed the touch." She clasped my hands in hers and looked into my eyes. "I can't know something until I get the feel of it. I bet you're the same."

An *aha* feeling sank down to my tailbone and made a home for itself.

"There will always be more to learn, grasshopper," the instructor said with a smile and a twinkle. "There will always be a deeper place to go, another layer of the onion to be peeled. So just give yourself a little more time."

❋

That day a seed was planted, a seed that would eventually grow into the unraveling of my belief that I had to be perfect in order to be loved.

How freeing!

From that seed my ego-self grew to learn there is no such thing as static perfection, only an organic process of learning. My job was to recognize my unique style and give it the time and space to grow.

It took a while, but the weight of needing to be perfect — or instantly knowledgeable — dissipated, allowing me to reintroduce innocence into my life. This in turn helped me to give up expecting myself to know (or not know) everything that someone else knew. And that, in turn, opened me up to what was really there. In other words, I began to learn how to *just be.*

We are like plants, taking time and attention to grow. We cannot be flowers before we have gone through the process of nourishing our seedlings. Why should we expect to be at the end of the learning curve before we have stepped into the beginning?

What is important is staying in Beginner's Mind, not allowing our past judgments or future expectations to impede our unique learning style and pace. Each way of processing information has a different combination of strengths and weaknesses — one is neither better nor worse. The key is to remain innocent.

Beginner's Mind facilitates the process of learning by allowing the knowledge to unfold in its own time without taking the wrong turns associated with premature judgments of how we think something *ought* to be. When we adopt the innocence of a beginner, 100 percent of our attention is focused in the present moment instead of having part of our minds time-traveling into the past or future. It doesn't matter whether we are artists or lawyers, plumbers or housewives, Beginner's Mind will help anyone suspend past judgments and be in the *here and now*.

As you read this book, allow yourself, once again, to be a beginner.

CHAPTER THREE

Having It All!

We are living, organic pieces of art — the sum total of all that we have experienced in life. Art in motion — forever opening and contracting, forever changing shape and expression. Like the dabs of color a painter applies, our experiences are imprinted on our body/mind. As we learn and grow we constantly rework our painting or refine the contours of our sculpture. A dab of paint here and a little shaving off there, but instead of a paintbrush or a chisel we use a different kind of tool: *feelings*. We have been molded, the way a sculptor molds clay, by each and every feeling we have ever had. The longer we live, the more we become a living map of our life's journey.

If we want to add a new road to our map — to change our living work of art — we cannot simply walk down the same old path or use the same old material. In order to live a different life, we are called to change the quality of the medium with which we create our organic piece of art. But because every cell holds the emotional memory of our past experiences, we need to go beyond our body, beyond our cells, beyond even our DNA to create something new. In fact, we need to go into a different art supply store altogether for new material to integrate into our old sculpture or painting. This art store is transcendental and is open all hours, every day of the week, from the beginning of time to the end of time. It supplies only one material. But this one material is infinitely versatile and of the purest quality. And with it we can do just about anything. If we knew how to get it, then... *we could have it all!*

Having it all, however, does not mean what many of us think it means. If we believe advertising, having it all means a well-paid job, a beautiful home filled with all the latest gadgets, a new car, and perhaps a holiday or two a year. Owners of corporations, in their bid to make money, bombard us with myriad choices that promise to make us happy. But what many of us are finding is that when we reach this goal of a better lifestyle, we are still not fulfilled. Many in our culture have had the privilege of going down this road of consumerism; to our surprise we have found that the much-touted idea of having it all does not ultimately make us *feel* happy.

Expecting to find happiness and contentment by acquiring objects doesn't work because consumerism is based on the belief that we do not have enough. We always need more clothes, a new sofa, a bigger house, a second or third car — all to keep us distracted from the truth of our situation, that we feel powerless. We think we are victims of disease, of bosses and their whims, of government, of terrorism, of banks, of family obligations, of dysfunctional relationships and our aging bodies.

What having it all means to me is a very different thing. To me, it means being Hooked-Up, exuding a sense of lightness, traveling through the world unburdened and connected to the flow of the Life Force. When we exude light, we create a wholly different work of art than we have been conditioned to create. Our experiences and feelings increase in depth and breadth. Our senses become keener. We open ourselves to the robustness of life. Our pain, grief, and disappointment simply become other colors on the palette of light.

If only we were conscious of the flow of the Life Force. If only we could access it at will — oh, how our lives would change! The current of lightness would carry us toward who we were meant to be, who our souls would naturally become.

To consciously experience light is not to go skipping down the road bellowing Broadway show tunes (though feel free if that's your fancy). Instead, to experience light is to allow into our conscious lives the energetic component that runs throughout the universe, and therefore throughout our body/mind. *Light* is merely a word. Some might substitute *peace* or *bliss*. Others, *gratitude*. Whatever word we put to it, what counts is the feeling of the energetic component when we are wholly in the present moment.

That's the key: the present moment. From the perspective of this energetic flow, the past and the future do not exist. There is just the ever-unfolding present. Anything else is an imaginary construct of the mind. While there's some usefulness in our imagined constructs, these constructs can impede our ability to truly focus on the present moment. If we could learn how to be in the present moment, we would have conscious access to this energetic flow.

The Relative and the Absolute

Maharishi Mahesh Yogi, the developer of Transcendental Meditation, says that when we are in the present moment we simultaneously recognize both aspects of the universe:

- the relative part that constantly changes, and

- the absolute part that never changes.

This absolute part is the origin of the energetic component, of that flow of light, of bliss, of peace and appreciation. It is where potential lives — the place from which all of creation springs. And it is what we often ignore.

We forget that everything is made of energy. The chair you are sitting on, this book you are reading, the car you drive in, the trees outside, the sky, and, of course, your body — all of these have their source in this absolute aspect of the universe.

To illustrate how this is true, let's look at a sample body. It is, say, six feet tall, 190 pounds, with brown hair, a medium build, and blue eyes. This body is a *relative* aspect of creation, which means we can touch it, see it, taste it, smell it, and hear it move through space. When we step nearer to this body and observe it closely, we see that the texture of the skin is smooth except for the fingertips and soles of the feet, the hair has a soft, fine texture, and on the left shoulder there is a mole.

When we look at this body under a microscope, we see that it is made of cells. These cells aren't worried about being late for work or what movie they want to watch that evening.

They are concerned about manufacturing chemicals and duplicating themselves and stopping invaders such as viruses, antigens, and bacteria. When we go even deeper, we see that these cells are made up of molecules. Molecules constitute the smallest quantity that a substance can be divided into without losing its characteristics. On this level it is hard for anyone who does not study chemistry to differentiate between the molecules of a human body and the molecules of a cat or a dolphin (or any other life form, for that matter).

Taking our observation further in, we see that a molecule is made up of two or more atoms. An atom is the smallest particle of an element that can exist and take part in a chemical exchange and still retain its identity. Atoms are composed of still smaller particles called electrons, neutrons, and protons. Comparatively speaking these small particles move around in a huge vacant territory. From this view we appear to be almost entirely made up of empty space. This view of the universe looks very different from the global view of our sample body. Now, it is even harder to differentiate between a body and anything else in creation.

Let's look still further, beyond the subatomic level. Here, elementary particles display very different laws of nature and can zip in and out of our perception. From this perspective there are no boundaries. We can't discern which particle comes from the human body or which comes from a rock, a cat, a star, a chair, or anything else. These particles sit on the threshold of emptiness and vibrate faintly, seemingly at random. Some vibrations die off to nothingness, while others manifest into our reality as energy. When they wink out of existence, where do they go? They drop down to a point of zero vibration, their source, the starting point. This starting point is common to everything that has ever been or will ever be created. From here there is no differentiation; everything is one and the same.

Maharishi Mahesh Yogi calls this place the *Unified Field*. It is the origin of the energetic flow that runs not only through the universe but also through our body/mind. It supports everything. And it feels light, like bliss, like peace, like gratitude infused throughout our being. From the perspective of the Unified Field there is only one of us.

※

I first learned about the Unified Field — and the meaning of the saying "We are all One" — during the late 1960s and early '70s. This was a time of reformation. Consciousness was shifting. Historically this was a pivotal moment when the Western world moved into a *New Age*. The Vietnam War was raging, the sexual revolution was blossoming, the music industry was forging new ground, and creativity was at a high. People were no longer satisfied with the status quo. We were discontented with the way things were and fearful over what the future might bring; we therefore doubted what we called "the establishment," and all that it stood for. We started to question everything: Is war necessary? Why can't I have long hair if I want it? Why do I get paid less just because I am a woman? Do I really need a bigger house and a new car?

For me, the first step toward expanding my consciousness and understanding the Unified Field was more ego based than spiritual. Late in the Calgary summer of 1969, I sat enthralled in a booth at Verona's Pizza Parlour. Chin in hand, elbow on the table, I drank in the words of my school friend as he expounded upon the virtues of Transcendental Meditation, or TM, as he called it. Like the zealous new initiate he was, he told me that all I had to do was meditate twice a day and enlightenment would be mine. I would become anchored in the light of profound knowledge; free from all worries and fears, I would appreciate the totality of life.

As I sat there listening to my friend, I realized I didn't have a clue about what he really meant by "profound knowledge" or "the totality of life," I just knew I wanted to be the one doing the telling, creating awe and envy in my fellow listeners. I had to learn how to meditate so I could walk around with that air of mystery, knowing I knew something that perhaps you didn't, or if you did that we were part of an elite club. As a result, late that August I was initiated into TM. It was the cool thing to do.

I began watching and listening to videotapes and audiotapes of Maharishi Mahesh Yogi, the developer of the TM technique, and after finding that they made incredible sense to me, both intellectually and intuitively, I knew I was on the right path, cool or not. I dutifully practiced TM twice a day. During these sessions I sat comfortably with my eyes closed, using the special sound or mantra I received at my initiation to help my mind turn inward. My thoughts became more and more subtle, taking me into a deep, warm, safe place filled with light that went beyond thought to the source of everything — the Unified Field.

To get there I had to let go, give up trying, use no effort. My first conscious experience of the Unified Field occurred not long after my initiation. I sat quietly, following the technique I had been taught, when all of a sudden a curtain opened in my perception. No matter where I looked in my mind's eye, I could see *nothing*; it was like sitting in the middle of a flat, sandy desert. I felt larger than the confines of my skin, with no boundaries, no walls, no gates, no scenes, no immediate thoughts. I also experienced a profound *feeling* of lightness, stability, and appreciation. I felt I had arrived home after a long journey through storms and floods and battles.

Twice a day every day, in my meditation my mind would dip into the unbounded reservoir of the Unified Field. I was completely at rest yet totally alert. I was still. I felt light. My mind was naturally drawn to these levels of greater and greater bliss just as our minds naturally wander to beautiful music wafting through an open window.

My ability to stay in the present moment and appreciate my surroundings increased the more I experienced my source. The more present I was, the more conscious I became of the source in all things — an enjoyable feedback loop. In this way I gradually gained a degree of awareness of the absolute quality of life in my everyday environment, which resulted in changes that went beyond my limited beliefs and enhanced my reality.

Since we can't experience the Unified Field without it directly affecting our relative existence, these experiences had far-reaching effects on me. Although I knew that deep down I was changing for the better, I really didn't know how much and how quickly this path would transform me. About four years after starting TM, I woke up to the realization that familiar parameters no longer existed. I felt, for a time, as if I were sliding down an icy slope with no brakes.

I looked around. I was living in foreign territory. A place unknown.

My entire perception changed. I dropped down into an even deeper level of experience. Nothing so far in my life had prepared me for the realizations that came with it. Words such as *still* and *contentment* took on new meaning. I came to understand them to indicate a profound sense of inner tranquility. And color wasn't something to just look at anymore; it had texture and sound and purpose. Green became a soft healing melody in a forest; red, a fiery, passionate storm. Everything I saw, touched, smelled, or heard had more depth and breadth. I perceived the underlying unity in all things. It was now obvious to me that the universe was a unique expression of our common source — the Unified Field.

I felt excited but also very scared as my old foundation started to crumble. Who I was and why I was here changed so quickly that I remember repeating to myself almost daily, "So this is who I am!"

And my outer world changed too. My marriage to my childhood sweetheart abruptly ended, and I moved across the country to Kingston. I wanted to ensure that I was not just paying lip service to a theoretical spiritual ideal. I wanted to walk my talk. At the time, the TM Organization was planning to build an academy nearby, and my intuitive sense encouraged me to seek this new idyllic setting in order to contemplate "life, the universe, and everything." At age twenty-four, I left my husband, my mother, my brother, my sister (who was my confidante), my friends, and my life as I knew it.

I started again.

Experiencing the Unified Field

Does this mean we have to practice Transcendental Meditation and start a new life to experience the Unified Field? Of course not. There are many ways to get acquainted with our source. TM just happened to be my first. But it does mean that when we regularly experience the Unified Field in a conscious way, we will give up life as we know it. For something better.

Bringing our awareness of the Unified Field into our daily life will cause all unsupportive aspects, such as the wrong job or dysfunctional mental/emotional habits, to become so obvious we will feel compelled to change them in order to feel better. Take heart, though; we can trust in this new direction because the Unified Field is intelligent.

This intelligence is expressed in the active component of the Unified Field — the Life Force. The results of this force are creative yet orderly. A seed becomes a seedling and grows into a beautiful mature plant. A tree is not created fully matured only to regress to being an acorn. When we plant a flower seed, we don't get a Dodge minivan. We aren't born with bark for skin or seaweed for hair. Because we recognize this basic principle, we can be assured that the Life Force will lead us to become more than we are right now.

For example, I *knew* when I left Calgary for Kingston that no matter what I encountered on my journey across the country, I was in the process of experiencing something greater than I had before. I trusted this growth in the same way I trusted the sun would rise in the east the next morning — and set in the west come evening. I understood I was an expression of that transcendental art store, the Unified Field, and its sole material, the intelligent energetic flow called the Life Force.

At any time we can feel the lightness of the Life Force by bringing our awareness to the present moment — that is, by consciously focusing on both sides of our existence: 100 percent on the relative and 100 percent on the absolute.

The relative aspect, which we perceive with our senses, follows rules such as gravity, time, and space. It is always changing, constantly moving from one form to another. When we observe a tree, we see the trunk, the leaves, and maybe some roots. We can smell its scent and touch the rough bark. The leaves change with the seasons; we can see and touch them as they change from green to gold to red. The bark and trunk change too, even though we cannot see it. The trunk grows a new ring each year, the growth reflecting the kind of year it had — its own personal map. In time the tree will die and form compost, just as our body goes through its life cycle and ages and eventually dies.

What we don't see at first glance is the source of our body or the tree — the part of life energetically rooted in the Unified Field; nevertheless, throughout all this growth and change, the source, the absolute, remains the same. It is the never-changing aspect of our life, the only constant we will ever experience. Whether we are happy or sad, sick or healthy, rich or poor, the common denominator in all of these scenarios is that we are *being* something. The *being* part is perennial. It is always there, rooted in our communal energetic reservoir, the Unified Field, and its active component, the Life Force.

From the time of my earliest memories, a quiet consistent feeling/voice has spoken to me, often manifesting itself as intuition. It has been a constant companion and has never changed its tone or peaceful presence no matter what the circumstances. This consistent feeling/voice, however, is not merely a part of me; it is my core, my Spirit, my energy signature, the central thread around which the rest of my life is woven. And it is through our Spirit or energy signature that we connect with one another and with the rest of creation. For example: We walk down a road on a beautiful day and we feel grateful. We look at our partner and we feel love. We touch our mother's hand and we feel safe. We hear a bird's song and we feel carefree. A spectacular sunset gives us a feeling of awe. These feelings are a manifestation of the energetic connection that underlies such moments in time — light meeting light, Spirit meeting Spirit — in the present moment.

This energy connection fuels us. With practice, we find it empowers us. It enables us to make clear, significant choices that lead to healthy life changes. Through this mindful connection we cease being victims reacting to circumstances but rather become creators of the life we want. Yes, by being consciously connected to our source we can have it all: the strength and self-empowerment to thrive as well as to enjoy the bounty around us.

Right here, right now.

Recognizing the Life Force

When we begin seeking the Life Force, we often find it is not always recognizable in obvious or superficial places. But it is everywhere. It is nonlocal energy unconfined to a single space/time, yet it has a measurable influence. At first the Life Force appears soft, quiet, subtle, and still, but only because we have been raised to focus on activity. While we are engaged in the intellectual navigation of our life, the Life Force fades into the background. When we learn to decrease our level of activity and quiet our minds, the Life Force suddenly appears everywhere. But in reality it hasn't changed; it has always been everywhere. Only our ability to recognize it has increased. By becoming present and letting go of our preoccupations, we effortlessly Hook-Up to it.

For example, imagine admiring a healthy newborn baby girl. Our first reaction might be to notice her soft, curly hair, blue eyes, and button nose. And who in the family has those funny toes? But at the same time, as our eyes and ears are drinking in all the *relative aspects*, we experience a feeling of wonder, of joy. Therein lies the Life Force. Therein lies the feeling of light. A newborn, relatively speaking, has no emotional baggage, no agenda, no pressure to perform. It is never in a rush but in a state of constant discovery. Such purity allows us to perceive the uncluttered Life Force as it is manifested through a living being.

It is found...in the pause.
In the wonder.
In the innocence.
It is behind whatever color looks good to us.
Behind whatever sound is soothing to our ears.
Between the notes of a melody.
Between our in-breath and our out-breath.
Behind whatever texture gives us pleasure and comfort.

It is behind a beautiful sunset and a rainy day.
It   is   found   in   the   spaces   between
these   words.
Behind a great painting.
Underneath our movement.
Between the cells in our body.
Inside the core of a tree.
It is still.
It is real.
It is here, now.

Being Present

In Zen Buddhism it is said that when we walk, we walk, and when we eat, we eat. Being present means our attention will not be on what happened to us last night or last year, or what we will be doing next month, or, for that matter, what we are going to have for dinner. We cannot be present while we are carrying a grudge against someone or when we are preoccupied with a current life crisis. Showing up, or being present, means that all of our attention is on the object or task at hand. There are numerous ways to find presence, many requiring at least one or two hours a day devoted to practice.

"But I just don't have the time!"

How often have you said these very words? One of the ways we lose our ability to respond to the question "How can I *feel* better?" is our sense that we just don't have the luxury of time to ponder and seek out new relationships with ourselves or with a higher purpose. Maybe that great job we were so happy to get required more overtime than we had anticipated. Maybe our children's needs became even more demanding as they navigated the labyrinth of their unique lives. Or as our parents aged it became payback time as they required more of our assistance to carry out their daily routine.

"There's just no time!"

But let's not throw out the baby with the bathwater. Take a deep breath. We're not talking about neglecting our responsibilities here. On the contrary, by putting our awareness in the present moment we not only experience a sense of lightness, but we are also more effective and have greater long-term productivity.

When we are not being present two problems occur: First, we no longer receive all the information available. Second, we separate ourselves from our fuel — the Life Force. Both create *dis-ease* and disharmony in our body/mind and upon the earth.

Instead, we need to educate and strengthen our nervous systems to accept the life-sustaining energy we require to thrive. The process of educating and strengthening our nervous systems by consciously reconnecting our Spirit to our physical self is, however, more than an intellectual construct. Real neuropeptides are unplugging from real receptor sites and plugging into new receptor sites, causing change on fundamental levels. The way to start this process is to *become present.*

Be careful, however, not to make becoming present a goal you must work hard for. Life is not about the destination; it is about the journey. Goals are great to set direction, but in order to implement them (contrary to cultural beliefs) it is best to relax into the present moment where the Life Force resides. To continuously focus on the goal jettisons us into the future, dividing our attention, taking us out of the here and now.

When I started to write this book I set a goal of having it finished in two years. That was five years ago! Staying focused on the goal and pushing myself forward to obtain it did not serve me because when I didn't stay in the present moment I couldn't access my creativity. I needed to Hook-Up to the Life Force (our source of creativity) and then stay in the present moment to allow this book to unfold one word, one paragraph, one page at a time.

Yes, we all intend to reach our goals, and we use that feeling of intention as an impetus to steer us through our life's journey. But the act of continually looking into the future or remembering the past is counterproductive. If our attention is on yesterday, or tomorrow, or last year, or twenty years from now, then we cannot be present. We cannot feel the quality of the absolute permeating the relative, right here and now. It is in the process, not the goal, that we find a fulfilling life. We set our intent or goal and then show up in the present moment to experience the process along the way.

There is no use telling yourself you will be happy when you retire. Allow yourself to be happy now. There is no use telling yourself you will practice being present after you finish the next contract, or after your children have grown and are on their own. When we stand in the present moment and perceive the relative aspect of our life along with the absolute (the Life Force of the Unified Field), we experience feelings of lightness, bliss, and peace in a real, tangible way. This is *having it all.*

CHAPTER FOUR

Trusting the Life Force

The Life Force is intelligent; I cannot say this enough. Although a body/mind may be jammed with impediments to the natural flow of the Life Force, it flows nevertheless. And despite the fact that our interpretation of the Life Force may be skewed, we can still trust that the source of this energy is all-knowing.

When I talk about the Life Force flowing through our bodies, I am essentially talking of emotion (that is, energy in motion, or E-motion). Unfortunately, many of us lack a clear understanding of our emotions and the ways in which our emotions operate in the body/mind. Further, our culture discounts emotions, considering them relatively unimportant, believing the intellect to be superior.

In modern Western culture many of us believe we can *think* our way into good decisions: If only we had enough information, enough data, we could fix our spouses, our children, our chronic headache, or our back pain, just as we fix a computer. We want the intellect to solve everything. And although the intellect plays an essential role in our overall makeup, it has many limitations. Where the intellect shines is in solving problems with its logical, linear way of organizing thoughts and ideas.

However, it has been my experience that many of the important aspects of life are nonlinear. Our relationships with one another (not to mention our relationships with ourselves) are often paradoxical, conflicting, and self-contradictory. The course of our life can change as a result of a seemingly random event: What would my life have turned into if I hadn't met my zealous TM friend at Verona's Pizza Parlour? It would have been quite different, I assure you. Can we really be surprised that most of us are not where we expected to be when we were young? The road that at first appeared as straight as an arrow turned crooked and labyrinthine.

Accepting that much of life is nonlinear can be a frustrating exercise for our intellect, because it must accept that it cannot extrapolate the ultimate consequences of any event, whether it appears at first to be good or bad. To attempt to judge the consequences can only be a delusion that ignores the fact that the process of nature is not based on a straight line but on the path of least resistance, which is an organic process, a continuous network of immense diversity. For this reason, it is wise to pay attention to the Life Force for guidance. It has the ability to navigate the nonlinear, to take us beyond our limited perception.

To illustrate, let me tell you a fable: Late one year a Colorado rancher lost his horse; during a storm it bolted into the mountains. Neighbors from an adjoining farm came around and said, "That's too bad." The rancher said, "Maybe." A day later, after the storm had cleared and the sky was bright and sunny, the horse came back, bringing five wild stallions with it. Upon hearing the news, the neighbors telephoned and said, "Isn't that great?" And the rancher replied, "Maybe." The next week, while attempting to tame the biggest of the stallions, the rancher's son broke his leg in three places. At the hospital, the neighbors who had come to visit shook their heads and said, "Well, that's just too bad, ain't it?" And the rancher said, "Maybe." The next day a letter of conscription arrived in the mail, requiring the son to fight in Vietnam, but he couldn't because of his broken leg. The same neighbors came around in the evening and said, "Isn't that wonderful?" And our rancher just said, "Maybe."

Our intellect cannot be an effective guide through life. The only guide worth its salt, the only guide able to answer anything other than "maybe" to a situation, is the Life Force, flowing out from the Unified Field through our Spirit and into our body/mind. It knows the shortest, most efficient path to our dreams. This is why, in our heart of hearts, in the core of our being, we long to be led by this force, living truly in the present moment.

❦

Let me tell you what happened to one of my editors. Rather than trusting in the guidance of the Life Force, she put an overemphasis on intellectual thought.

We arranged to meet at a café called Serious Coffee on a Wednesday morning for a not-so-serious cup of tea — and to review the edits she had done on my manuscript. I got there early, chose a table facing the window to take advantage of the sunny day, took off my jacket, hung it around my chair, and went to the counter to place my order. Going back to the table, I glimpsed my editor's back as she bent to pay a cab driver.

Odd, I thought. *Where's her red scooter?*

Juggling her shoulder bag, two plastic grocery bags, and a large manila envelope containing what I guessed was my manuscript, my editor walked the few steps to the café doors and fumbled with the handle. Just as I realized she could use a helping hand, she burst through the door. My eyes immediately fell upon the reason for her cab ride and flustered behavior — she had a cast on her right hand that went halfway up her arm. I took her grocery bags and the envelope (which was indeed my manuscript) and helped her take off her black and yellow coat.

Plopping into a chair and unwinding her yellow silk scarf from around her neck, my editor let out a big sigh, ran her good hand through her cropped gray hair, looked up into my face, and said, "Tea first, story later."

Taking her order to the counter, I was back with her tea in record time. I leaned my elbows on the table. "So . . . what happened?"

"Well," she began, sinking back into her chair with another sigh, "last Saturday night my niece invited me out to that new *Charlie's Angels* flick. I'd slept badly the night before — hot flashes kept me up half the night. You know what that's like?"

"*Moi?*" I said, mimicking innocence. "I have no idea what

it's like to get so hot I could fry an egg on the top of my head every twenty minutes."

Smiling now, she carried on. "As usual I was up with the birds, feeling much worse than a refried egg, sort of like a fried running shoe, an old, worn-out one with tattered laces. I tried to nap in the afternoon but couldn't seem to settle down. So, when it came time to go to the movie, all I wanted to do was crawl under my new yellow duvet with a good book. But no. I had made a commitment to my niece, and now I *had* to honor it. Last time we were supposed to get together, I canceled, so I couldn't disappoint her again. I pulled myself together as best I could and went off on my scooter."

"So how was the movie?" I asked, taking a sip of Earl Grey.

"Unbelievably loud and in my face; it wore me out. Drained me completely. My niece had a great time at least, so that counts for something. Afterward, I struggled to keep a smile on my face while saying good-bye. How I managed the two blocks back to my scooter is a mystery. All I kept feeling was my yummy yellow comforter around me.

"As I reached the parking spot where I left my scooter, a black monster of a truck pulled up and a big burly man with beady eyes leaned out his window and asked in a gruff voice, 'You leavin'?' Only his question sounded more like a demand. I had to look up past his thick, shiny brute of a chrome grill to answer, 'Of course. As soon as I can.' I almost put a *Sir* at the end of it. But, instead of waiting, the guy edged his truck forward before I'd even sat down! Scared now, I jumped on my scooter. Turned the ignition. And zoomed off. In my rush, though, I forgot I'd been having trouble with my throttle: Just as I rounded the corner to Yates Street, the motor revved. The bike slid. I lost control. It fell on my hand. I heard a crack but pushed the implication of it away."

I nodded in empathy. "Good grief! Didn't anyone stop to help you?"

"Oh, it all happened much too fast for that. I didn't stop to feel; I just reacted. Cars zoomed past. I hauled the bike upright and pushed home. Not till I arrived did I allow myself a peek at my feelings. As soon as I did, I burst apart in a geyser of tears. I wailed and berated myself. If only I had listened to my feelings in the first place! Now my hand was a mess. It throbbed like crazy!"

She squirmed in her chair at the memory. "I knew I needed to go to the hospital but couldn't get up the energy. I just couldn't! Instead I popped some pain pills and fell asleep. A few hours later — it must have been around two — I woke up in excruciating agony. I knew, without a doubt, that I had broken a bone. After four hours in the emergency room, with the birds up and singing again, I finally crawled under my warm yellow duvet and got the rest I had so desperately needed in the first place."

"Wow. How is your hand now?"

"It still throbs a little," she said as she held her plaster cast up and gently wiggled her fingers, "but it's much better than it was." Placing her hand slowly back in her lap, she took a sip of her herbal blend and reached for the large manila envelope.

❊

My editor's conditioning dictated her decision to go to the movies, a common occurrence. We often have to contend with multiple emotional currents when we're making decisions. My editor was faced with deciding either to listen to her emotions of guilt (Life Force energy translated by past beliefs) or her bodily sensations of wanting rest (Life Force energy translated by her cells). If, before she went to the movies, my editor had taken a few moments to bring her attention to the present moment and use Beginner's Mind, she probably would have made a different decision.

Stated in this way, with hindsight, it may not seem too tricky to make a decision, but while navigating what at the time seems like myriad emotional energies, it is easy to go astray. Here is a quick rule of thumb: The choice that aligns us with our Spirit, our central thread leading back to the Unified Field, is the choice that elicits a *feeling* of lightness, bliss, and peace. If neither choice elicits such an emotion, then choose the one that comes closest.

Mentastics 1:
Discerning the Origin of Your Emotions

1. Bring to mind a situation in which you have to make a choice between one thing and another. It can be an important choice or one as benign as what to make for dinner.
2. Close your eyes if you can. (If you are driving, keep your eyes open!) Take a couple of easy, deep breaths into your chest and belly.
3. Imagine making one of the possible choices (for example, going to see *Charlie's Angels*).

4. Imagine following through with that choice (for example, meeting your niece, walking up to the theater, hearing the music, tasting the popcorn...). Don't put your vision in a box; allow innocence to enter.

5. Now imagine the event over, the task complete, the movie finished. Make it as visceral as you can.

6. How do you feel? What label(s) would you use to describe the energy running through your body?

7. Now pause and shake your body out. That's right; get up and be like a swimmer warming up before a race. Gently shake those limbs; neutralize that biochemistry.

8. Your next step is to imagine the alternate scenario. Get into it (for example, curling up with your yellow duvet). Don't assume what it will be like. Use Beginner's Mind. Put yourself into the situation and allow it to unfold.

9. Imagine the scenario afterward. Give yourself permission to bring the sensations right into your body.

10. How do you feel? How would you describe the energy moving through your body?

11. Okay. Do the swimmer warm-up shake; gently shake your limbs.

12. To the best of your knowledge and experience, which feeling is most like lightness, like bliss, like peace?

The point here is to get in touch with how we *feel* about a situation, not whether some agenda is fulfilled. Whichever decision results in a *feeling* more like bliss, like peace, like lightness is the one most closely aligned with our Spirit — whether our intellect can make sense of it or not!

Please do not interpret this to mean that just because we may not want to chop our wood or carry our water that we shouldn't. We all have to earn our crust of bread. But if we want our career and daily grind to change, we need to bring ourselves to the present moment. No matter what we are doing, we will do it better and carry less of a burden if we decide to Hook-Up to the Life Force, where the intelligent energy of our Spirit can carry and guide us.

Part of what distracts us from this support and guidance are our past expectations. Virtually all of us have already set up automatic agendas by assuming what our recurring experiences will be like. We have thrown expectations forward from the past into the future. And now, when we attempt to show up in the present moment, they miraculously reappear, getting in the way.

We do this all the time: We assume how a situation — work, let's say — will unfold. We just *know* we'll have a rotten time at that lousy job. The boss will jump down our throats. The clients won't return our phone calls. Our coworkers will be petty and self-serving, as usual.

In the same way we pigeonhole ourselves. We assume how we will respond to our spouse, our children, the homeless on the street, the stranger on the bus, the hunk at the bar. We are absolutely sure of it. On and on our assumptions go, keeping us in a box, chasing our tails round and round. With such strong, premeditated assumptions, finding our Spirit can sometimes seem like searching for a golden needle in the proverbial haystack.

But take heart. While it is true that not being in presence in the past makes it harder to be in presence now, it is also true that being in presence now will make it easier to be in presence later. It is like putting money into a compounding interest account: Presence grows. The more we are in presence now, the less expectations and assumptions will blindside us in the future. A few moments of presence every day will blossom exponentially in the future. So relax. Loosen up. *Trying* is counterproductive when entering the present moment. Apply Beginner's Mind instead. There is no pressure. A drop here, a drop there will become buckets later on.

Presence is a seed we sow. Water it. Be patient. And watch it grow.

CHAPTER FIVE

Clear Communication

Like attracts like. Birds of a feather flock together. The same is true of the energy we send out to the world. The quality of our life — from our bank account to our relationships — correlates to the quality of our feelings. Like feelings attract like situations. It's the nature of the universe. Each one of us is like an electromagnet, our fields interacting with every other field, attracting toward us situations of the same flavor as our emotions.

Empowered people come together. Loving people find others who love. Successful people connect. Unsuccessful people hang out with unsuccessful people. Emotionally wounded people form relationships with others of similar ilk. A man who is angry finds injustice everywhere he looks. A waiter in a bad mood doesn't attract tippers. A car saleswoman depressed from her slump doesn't attract buyers. Like attracts like.

This isn't a new concept. Many of us have read about it,

and all of us have experienced the power of our emotions firsthand: When we feel good, things tend to go well; when we don't feel good, things tend to go from bad to worse.

How are we to bring our emotions under control? How can we tailor our emotional energy to get us the results we want? Reasonable questions, but the hard part is not asking them! These questions are in themselves flawed. The very idea of controlling or "tailoring" our emotions implies manipulation. Manipulation — *trying* to make ourselves feel a certain way, perform a certain way, *be* a certain way — is, at best, a short-term fix, a Band-Aid. Manipulation is ego-centered, giving our intellect control. How can our ego-self know what lies beyond its safe little box?

What we want is to give our Spirit control. When we do this, we allow the genuine and authentic energy of our Spirit (lightness, bliss, peace) to come through. To do this, we don't try to control; we release into the present moment and effortlessly allow the wisdom of the Life Force to guide our journey. Consider what a joy life will be when we consciously radiate such Spirit energy, such feelings, into our everyday life.

When we get a taste of this greater flow, our consciousness naturally wants more — and then more. Our consciousness always gravitates toward a clearer quality of flow, toward greater peace, more comfort, easier pathways. We can't help it; it's inherent in the nature of our consciousness.

Impediments and blockages to the Life Force in our body/mind soon become self-evident and unacceptable. As these impediments or blockages dissolve, a process of clearing unfolds. Just as when we flush water through a clogged pipe, bits of muck occasionally fly astray. This process of clearing can be simultaneously painful and rewarding, confusing and illuminating.

For this reason it is helpful to understand how the components of our body/mind work and interact with one another as this clearing process unfolds. And it will unfold — you can count on it! However, you can also count on being led to a place where living is light and effortless, where your dreams manifest with joy. The Life Force is intelligent, remember. If given a chance the Life Force will lead you to Spirit and the bliss of the Unified Field.

The components of our body/mind that we will discuss are our labels and beliefs, and their subsequent holding patterns in our body. Without understanding how these components influence our communication to and from Spirit, we will often find ourselves lost in a tangle of complexity. When we have a foundation of comprehension under our belt, we will be conscious enough to choose differently.

The Components

Our unconscious mind functions as a transmitter, a translator, and a filter between our conscious body/mind and Spirit. It is the go-between. Through our unconscious, the energy of the Life Force (E-motion, or energy in motion) is channeled. Interacting within our unconscious body/mind is an interconnected web of components, which are labels, beliefs, and their corresponding holding patterns.

If I could make the lines of communication linear from our conscious body/mind to the Unified Field, they would look something like this:

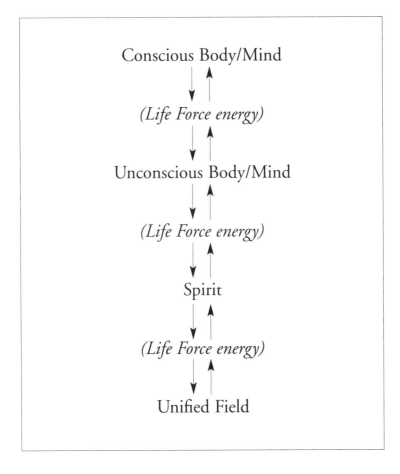

First, before we investigate the specific components lurk-
ing in our unconscious, let's take a look at the general manner in which the unconscious operates.

If we were an iceberg, our unconscious would be the 90
percent under the waterline. So if the tip of our iceberg (our
conscious body/mind) wants to go one direction, but the
part of us below the surface wants to go another, which carries more weight? You know it: Whichever way our unconscious wants to go is where we're going, regardless of how

much we stamp our feet in denial. Is it any wonder we feel powerless? When we understand the components operating within our unconscious and are able to clearly hear and follow the desires of our Spirit, we will find fulfillment.

Unfortunately, impediments or blockages in our unconscious body/mind often radically skew our interpretation and/or partially block the messages coming from Spirit. If our conscious body/mind is not consistently aware of Spirit in our life, it is because our unconscious has been conditioned to disregard the present moment, living through the past or the future.

This is what happened to my editor in the incident I shared with you. Her overzealous belief in commitment partially blocked her interpretation of the Life Force, allowing her intellect to make a decision she'd rather take back. Most of us run into such difficulties. We are pawns being controlled by our outdated and dysfunctional beliefs and postures.

Wouldn't it be great to choose more freely rather than reacting automatically? Of course it would. But first, before we can exercise mindful choices, it is helpful to understand the mechanics of the transmitter, the unconscious — that part of ourselves that creates and keeps our beliefs and postures in place.

Our Autopilot

Built into the unconscious is an automatic pilot. We do not consciously have to be aware of our hair growing, our blood flowing, our lungs breathing, our heart pumping, our eyes blinking; these things are automatic. Similarly, when trauma (either physical or emotional) enters our lives our unconscious sets up a mechanism to automatically deal with that event, causing the body/mind to compensate for the trauma. If this compensating posture is left in place, a holding pattern or repetitive way of being will form and therefore skew or disrupt the Life Force and our communication with Spirit.

A simple example of a physical holding pattern happened after my editor broke the bone in her hand. Her autonomic nervous system (under the direction of the unconscious) set up chemical reactions to cushion the break with a "plasma cocktail," which stiffened the surrounding muscles to hold the break in place.

My friend used her other hand to wash her hair, carry groceries, and chop vegetables so her fractured hand could heal. Later, after the break had healed, she continued to hold her hand in the same stiff manner — the unconscious was still operating in crisis mode and hadn't released the brakes. She did not direct her unconscious to let go, so her muscles carried on, holding themselves stiffly in this compensating posture even though their job had been done. On a very fundamental level, they had formed the *habit* of holding themselves rigid. Her hand forgot what it *felt* like to be supple, soft, and flexible.

This process also happens in the body after an emotional trauma. We have all been in confrontational situations: family conflicts, disagreements with angry co-workers, the death of a loved one. My editor friend experienced the emotional trauma that fear brings when the truck driver harassed her. In reaction to fear, her fight-or-flight impulse stimulated, she pulled away from the flow of the Life Force by stiffening her shoulders, tensing her lower back, and gritting her teeth as adrenaline surged through her body. Fear forced her to take off like a bullet and, combined with the forgotten faulty throttle, to lose control of her scooter. Even when the confrontation subsided, her unconscious did not forget. It retained the memory of her reaction so it could respond with the same pattern under future fearful situations.

This is how new postures get wired into the body/mind — unconsciously. Before long they become physical holding patterns, which powerfully distort our communication with Spirit and the Unified Field. It would not be an understatement to say that, to a large degree, such patterns dictate how clearly Spirit manifests in our bodies and in our lives; they are the part of us below the waterline.

From Labeling to Beliefs

Whether we are aware of it or not, the energy of the Life Force constantly flows through our bodies. Automatically, our brains tend to interpret the different ways in which this energy moves. Each way is given a label. This label is what we call a *feeling*.

When the energy that flows through our bodies is strong and comes in a rush accompanied by an aggressive thought, our brains might label this feeling as "anger." When the energy is impeded we might say we are "tired," or maybe "frustrated." And while we might name these kinds of experiences with the same label, it is a common misconception that everyone experiences the specific sensations of these energies in an identical way. Yes, there are often similarities — we all understand what anger means, or what tiredness means — but your specific experience of a particular feeling is *unique* to *you*.

To get a physical understanding, do the following mental gymnastics.

Mentastics 2: Feeling Energy Patterns

1. Close your eyes.
2. Let a feeling come to you. Are you feeling sad, angry, happy, anxious?
3. Think of a specific scenario that elicits this feeling. Visualize the scenario. Take your time. Be in the middle of the experience; breathe it in.
4. Where in your body is this feeling located? Is it in your chest, head, belly? What shape does it have? If this feeling had texture, what would it be? What color? Smell? Do not judge this energy. It only has the meaning we give it.
5. Start to play with it. Imagine it a different shape. How do you feel now?
6. Now imagine it a different color, a different texture. Check in. How would you define your feeling now?
7. Spread this energy as if you were pouring warm oil to encompass your whole body. Has your interpretation changed again?
8. Now imagine this energy pooling into nothingness at your feet, like water soaking into the ground.
9. Bring attention to your breath as it expands and contracts in your chest.
10. Gently open your eyes and notice how you feel.

The particular energy pattern you just recalled is what you labeled "anger" or "confidence" or whatever feeling you experienced. It was a single memory that related to a single feeling. *You* gave it that definition. *You* took that particular energy shape and called it something.

(If you haven't done the exercise yet, do it now and experience what I mean. In fact, let me go a step further and say that if you skip the exercises in this book you will miss much of the point, which is to have the *feeling* of Spirit, and ultimately the Unified Field, in your tissue and bones, not only in your mind.)

Labeling is neither good nor bad; it is simply the way our minds make sense of things. We use labels repeatedly as shortcuts to define energy patterns. They enable us to quickly interpret our emotions and respond to them while interacting in a variety of situations and environments.

Most often labels were set down when we were young. Think of it. When was the first time you experienced a feeling of loss? Age two? Three? Perhaps a little baby sister or brother came into the family and you lost the undivided attention of your parents. Emotion welled up inside your little tummy and formed into some shape, perhaps a hard lump. From that point on, that shape and texture, or anything resembling it, became defined in your unconscious as "loss."

Over time the recurring use of a label gets translated, consciously or unconsciously, into a belief. Like labels, beliefs are neither good nor bad; they are simply the way our minds organize the multiple, diverse, and interconnected feelings we have every moment of every day. Regardless of whether we are aware of them, beliefs organize our inner life, the part of us below the waterline. Because we generally hold on to our beliefs, they provide an intellectual continuity, guiding us, for better or worse, through both the calm and the choppy waters of our day-to-day existence. They define who we *think* we are, but not who we actually are. Who we really are is indefinable because we are not static. A belief, with its accompanying labels, implies that we will not change. In truth, we are living works of art, constantly being molded and changed as we experience life.

Beliefs are merely meanings we have placed on recurring E-motions, like naming paths that we frequently travel. Experiencing the same belief or energy pattern over and over again has a corresponding effect on the body because the mind is inseparable from the body. These repetitive pathways translate into our bodies as holding patterns. And these holding patterns can be helpful or detrimental depending on what's driving them.

Using the example of you as a child suddenly having a new sibling to contend with, you lost the undivided attention of your parents and experienced confusion, upset, and an emptiness in your belly, where your innocent trust used to be. This emptiness hurts, so your unconscious comes to the rescue and gathers that feeling into a lump to protect you. You welcome the lump — it has a good association because it eases your pain. Without that hard lump, you would hurt. Your belly, over time, gets used to the feeling of housing a hard ball; you feel safe with it there. The repeated experiences you have with this label soon become organized into a belief structure called "abandonment." You now believe that when your brother came along, your parents abandoned you in favor of him.

Not only does this belief have behavioral repercussions, but the automatic pilot button perpetuates the feeling of a hard lump in your belly as a coping mechanism every time you find yourself in similar circumstances: when your best friend moves away, when your pet dies, or when you lose a partner. Carrying the feeling of loss around in your belly on a constant basis can lead to many dysfunctional conditions, including indigestion, cramps, diarrhea, constipation, ulcers, and food sensitivities.

The components of labels, beliefs, and holding patterns form an interconnected web. Changing one influences them all. In the same way, they are self-perpetuating; each one reinforces the others.

❧

For a specific example that illustrates how these three elements work and relate to one another, let me tell you a story from my childhood.

My five-year-old finger reached up and pressed the brass bell. The door opened on well-oiled hinges. A smiling mouth on the serene face of a tall, elegant woman said, "Well, hello again; come on in."

A golden curl peeked out from behind the door, followed by laughing blue eyes. My playmate turned and ran down the hall, calling over her shoulder, "Follow me. I've got a surprise!"

Quickly laying my scuffed white sandals next to her shiny black patent leather Mary Janes, I ran along the hall's plush carpet and down the stairs into a basement playroom. My eyes, like two suns emerging from behind a cloud, lit up. "Wow!"

Giggling, my playmate's small hand lifted to cover her wide, bright smile. "My mom just got it for me."

Fabrics: reds and blues, yellows and greens, velvets, silks, cottons and leather — masses of them — overflowed onto her lap. A dress-up box: I had always wanted one.

My playmate jumped up, snapped closed the lid of the emptied antique trunk, stuck her regal nose in the air, and declared, "We shall be queens ruling over our subjects. Let us put on our gowns!"

As she pulled a glittery silver robe over her new yellow blouse, I rifled through the costume pile until I came upon a purple velvet coat. It fit generously, concealing my faded blue hand-me-down dress.

"We shall line up our subjects in front of our thrones," she declared in the same royal voice, "so we may hear their troubles and advise them."

I copied my playmate's tone. "Let us use the dolls." I stated, stroking my lavish turned-up sleeve as if it were a cat.

Our eyes turned to the golden-haired Princess Anastasia. She sat in her place of honor among her ladies in waiting in the middle of the top shelf. Gauzy peach fabric floated about her delicate body, highlighting the blush on her porcelain cheeks. Simultaneously, we both reached for her.

"*I* want to play with Anastasia!" I cried, pulling the doll my way.

"She's mine, and *I* get first choice," my friend shouted back, pulling the doll her way. A tug of war ensued. I doubled my efforts.

"I'm the guest so *I* get first choice!" And I yanked the doll right out of her hands.

My playmate's jaw clenched, her eyes narrowed into two slits, and her face broke into blotchy red spots. With the meanest look I'd ever seen and the loudest voice I'd ever heard, she shrieked, "You are the most *selfish* person in the whole wide world!"

My eyes widened. My shoulders rounded and scooted up to my ears. My cheeks burned with embarrassment. She was so intense; I felt she must be right. Was I selfish? No time to think about that; this confrontation threw me into defensive mode. I took a deep breath and shouted back: "Oh yeah! I saw her first. You didn't have to try to take her away. You always get to play with her."

My playmate's bottom lip trembled. Tears pooled in her eyes. "Princess Anastasia is my very best friend, the only one who makes my tummy better."

In response, my own tummy hardened like a coconut shell while my insides churned into sour milk. A lump congealed in the back of my throat. I tried to swallow it down. Tears welled.

I gave the doll back.

❖

I can write about this incident now as if I was conscious of the whole process at the time, but in truth most of this process took place below my waterline. From that point on, my behavior in my friend's basement became unconsciously defined in my young mind by the label "selfish." This label automatically elicited "shame," another label. In turn, both these labels became linked directly to an energetic pattern — the feeling of a hard nauseated belly and a lump in the throat. For years to come when I coveted something someone else wanted, an identical physical/emotional response would well up, reminding me I was selfish. Before I knew it, I had assumed the belief "I am inherently a selfish person," which I carried throughout the rest of my childhood and into adulthood.

This belief, with its labels and corresponding energetic pattern, became twisted into a tight bundle that I later chose to respond to with either defiance or generosity. I vacillated from selfishness (jutting out my chin and puffing up my chest to announce to the world that, no matter what, I was doing *this* for me) to selflessness (putting another's needs before my own to prove to the world, and myself, that I was *not* selfish).

In an attempt to diminish my feeling of nausea, my unconscious automatically reacted the same way it would react to a broken bone or damaged tissue: It stiffened the surrounding area to protect the trauma, in this case the muscles of my belly. In this way the stiffness stayed in place and formed a holding pattern that skewed my movement and subsequent communication with Spirit, leading to stomach difficulties later on. Over time, a hard belly became normal for me.

⁂

Our bodies and our minds are interconnected through the components of labels, beliefs, and holding patterns. Here is another story that looks at this interconnected web from the opposite direction — from the physical to the emotional.

It was a hot August evening. My family and I ambled along the dusty cracked sidewalk in small-town Saskatchewan. We were going to have a rare dinner out. My Dad, in one of his playful moods, licked his lips and quickly rubbed his hands together. "I can't wait! The Star Café has the best Denver sandwiches west of Portage La Prairie; their pickles are deee-licious," he muttered as if to himself, then slyly peeked to check if my older sister and I were paying attention.

"Can I have a Denver sandwich all to myself?" I pleaded, craning my neck to look up into his hazel eyes.

"Do you think you can eat a whole one?" he asked with a coy smile, a wisp of thin dark brown hair drifting onto his brow.

"Of course!" I promised, puffing out my chest. "I'm a big girl now; right, Momma?"

"Yes, you certainly are," she acknowledged from the rear, as she pushed my younger brother in his stroller.

Oh boy, for the first time my sister and I didn't have to share! We locked arms and skipped ahead, singing at the top of our lungs: "You are my sunshine, my only sunshine. You make me happy, when skies are gray…" The tiny white polka dots on my best pink dress caught my attention; the dots danced and jumped in time to our steps. Suddenly — splat! — I was facedown on the cement.

Abandoning my brother's stroller, my mother ran to pick me up. "How many times do I have to tell you to watch where you're going? Look at your dress; it's filthy," she scolded as she wiped bits of gravel and blood off me with a tissue from her purse.

"I'm sorry, Momma," I mumbled and hung my head to hide my tears. "I can't help it."

My father slowly shook his head. "What a clumsy girl you are!" he said, only he said it in Russian: *"Ech ti klatcha!* Every time I look at you, you're covered in scrapes and bruises. Don't you know how to walk yet? From now on, I'll call you *klatcha."*

And he did.

The name *klatcha* stuck, all the way into my adolescence and beyond. When I was in school, just walking down the hall or traversing the stairs was more than enough reason to trip. Embarrassed, I made jokes: "My flying lessons aren't going so well today," or "I got intimate with the floor tiles this morning."

This caused everyone to laugh and recite the standard reply: "Oh, you're such a *klatcha!"* With all this reinforcement, the feeling of being clumsy became fixed in my unconscious. There was no real conscious decision. I simply believed what people were telling me. I was clumsy; my family said so, my friends said so, and the scars on my hands and knees said so. It never occurred to me that I could be another way. As a result, my body/mind closed off new information regarding my body's ability to keep me upright.

Further, my clumsiness made me feel unbalanced. Over time, cautiousness became a way of being. Not only did I shy away from skiing, climbing, and running; I avoided any quick, strenuous movement as well. This shyness also bled into my emotional makeup. I was cautious about any kind of change. Planning in advance became a necessity. Last-minute changes were unwelcome — they knocked me off balance, made me flustered.

Not until my thirties did I discover the reason for my

clumsiness. It happened during a jazz dance class at the local Sportsplex. The instructor asked us students to stand in line with our feet parallel as she pranced up and down to inspect our posture. I stood as straight as I could, my head held high as I admired my reflection in the mirrored wall, but she immediately singled me out: "Your right leg isn't facing forward, dear."

I looked down. She was right. Even though my feet felt as if they were straight, they weren't. Strange. I had a misaligned right leg. It turned out forty-five degrees. How odd! Even though I'd tripped through life this far, I'd never noticed this before. My stance felt *normal* to me.

At home later, after cooking and serving dinner, cleaning up, and bathing and putting my two sons to bed, I took a moment for myself and plopped down on the couch with a cup of tea. My thoughts kept returning to the jazz class. The teacher's words made me wonder if being a *klatcha* was not inherent. Perhaps being easily knocked off balance was due merely to my misaligned leg. Maybe this trait was not set in stone, not irreversible. Maybe I could correct this. Choose differently. All my life I'd thought I was clumsy. I'd thought there was something intrinsically wrong with me. I was caught in the self-perpetuating loop of identifying with a belief that said, "This *klatcha* is me." But now, for the first time, as I sipped the last of the Earl Grey, I asked myself whether this label and its corresponding belief were perhaps only one possible interpretation. And could it be that my lack of emotional equilibrium was simply an extension of this interpretation? Could that be changed too? Could I really choose differently? *But how?* I wondered, placing the empty cup in the sink. How?

Getting Ready

This is a good question: How can we choose differently? But just as important as *how* is *what*. What would we choose differently if we could? Before we can choose something else, we need to know what that something else is. It is not enough to know what you *don't* want; you also need to know what you *do* want.

Okay, I wanted to stop identifying with the belief that said, "This *klatcha* is me." That's a good step. But what did I want to replace it with? Instead of feeling cautious and off balance, what did I want? I wanted to feel balanced and stable. I wanted to feel empowered, enthusiastic, passionate, creative, and abundant. I wanted to feel bliss. I wanted to feel light.

This may not seem like much of a revelation — that is, until we consider what most of us have been conditioned to want. We want the fancy red sports car and a house full of newfangled gadgetry. We want acreage in the country, or a cabin nestled in a forest clearing. We want a fragrant perennial garden, a view of the ocean, intimacy without conflict. And we want truckloads of money with the free time to spend it.

But, as I indicated earlier, those of us who have had the privilege of going down this road have found to our surprise that the blissful feelings that at first came with these objects soon faded. And we found ourselves searching once more for that scenario, that object, that would give us back our bliss. Over and over again we did this, searching for the next fix.

If we are honest with ourselves, however, all we ever really want is this feeling of bliss. It is never the objects or scenarios we want, but the feelings we associate with them. In the end, bliss and a sense of lightness are all we ever want. When the ride is over, there is nothing more important.

So, we want to feel blissful, light, at peace. That's a fairly generic statement. Some might even say cliché. But it's true, isn't it? I want to feel this way. My friends do too. So does my family. Cliché or not, deep down we all want to be at peace, to be blissful and light.

This feeling (or the lack thereof) can be our guide, our barometer that indicates to us where we are. Namely, in heaviness or lightness, in bliss or not in bliss. Bliss and a lightness of being are what flows from Spirit every second of every day of every year from the beginning to the end of time. The energy of the Life Force in its raw, pure form *is* light, unadulterated bliss. This is what we want, what our being naturally gravitates toward. And the present moment is where we access it.

Unfortunately, precious few of us are able to Hook-Up to the Life Force in the present moment. As a matter of fact, many of us would be hard-pressed to recall what bliss feels like in our body. To most, it is a foreign concept. Pie-in-the-sky nonsense.

This is our dilemma, the main reason why so many of us have so much difficulty choosing differently. If 99.9 percent of our bodies' experiences of the Life Force have registered after our beliefs and holding patterns have subdivided, criticized, analyzed, and sent the Life Force through a house of mirrors, turning it upside-down into fear, then the idea of bliss and light could sound understandably absurd. In one way or another we experience everything through our bodies.

As a result, if our bodies have no access, no memory, no experience of what it feels viscerally to be in the present moment, flowing with the unimpeded Life Force, then how can we choose it even if we know we want it?

This, in my experience, is where the Trager Approach is at its most powerful. It can transfer the feeling of the unimpeded Life Force into our tissue, our bones, our joints. And it can do so not only while we are in stillness, meditating, but also while we are in motion, driving a car, working, playing, making love. In this way Trager can help to recondition our bodies (and therefore our unconscious body/mind) to accept and remember the light and peaceful energy flowing to us from the Unified Field.

※

I was lucky. Although I had yet to be introduced to Trager, because of my years of meditation I had at least experienced what the Unified Field felt like. But what I was just beginning to understand, while drinking Earl Grey after my jazz dance class, was that, during the daily grind of motherhood — vacuuming and dusting the house, feeding and cleaning up after the kids — the bulk of me below the waterline was on autopilot, still following outdated and inaccurate directions from my childhood. Even though I knew I wanted the feeling of light, of bliss, of peace, my unconscious body/mind was hindering my efforts.

I tried to bully myself into changing, telling myself, *Stop it!* But that didn't work. I thought about ways I could manipulate my inner dynamics, use affirmations to train my unconscious to do my bidding. But such manipulative tactics were futile because they were giving control of my life to my intellect, my ego. And as we have discussed, the linear intellect is a poor guide.

What I needed to do was to put control of my life squarely in the hands of Spirit. So, I turned inward and asked Spirit to bring me what I needed. I asked without expectation. It was easy to adopt an innocent attitude since I was without any ideas of my own. I opened myself up to the possibility of something new and unexpected.

Serendipitously, a few weeks later while visiting friends in small-town Ontario, my husband and I were invited by our hosts to attend a demonstration of the Trager Approach given by a doctor friend of theirs. Simple curiosity made the four of us pile into the car and drive to the community hall. In front of a small crowd of about twenty, the enthusiastic doctor joyfully "danced" around her volunteer's body, jiggling his belly and rolling his head, tossing his limbs lightly in the air. As the demonstration progressed, I began to drool (inwardly of course). My body craved to be the one on the table. To my surprise I found I also yearned to be the one doing the dancing.

My body/mind quivered with joy. This was harmony in motion. This was exactly what I'd been looking for. I had found my next step. Trager.

❧

I made a series of appointments right off. Not with the enthusiastic doctor, mind you — she was, to my surprise, only an intermediate student — but with a seasoned practitioner.

During my first Trager session, while being interviewed by the practitioner, I related to her my revelation during my jazz dance class at the local Sportsplex.

"I have a belief that I am clumsy and easily knocked off balance," I said. "I think it is connected to my turned-out right foot. I keep affirming to myself that I'm not out of balance but that I'm instead exploring the strength of my center."

"Is it making a difference?" she asked.

"Not really."

"That's because you probably don't have a body experience of what it *feels* like to stand in your center, grounded and secure. The intellectual understanding is great. It gets you going in the right direction. Gets you searching. But our power to change comes from our feelings. And for that we must have an experience. Getting a feeling is like the measles; you catch it from someone who's got it."

As I undressed for the table portion of the session, keeping my underwear on, I noticed a poem that had been taped to the wall. It was words from Milton Trager:

> Not until we experience it
> Is it more than just words.

> After we experience it
> There is no need for words.

> The value of words
> Is to stimulate
> The desire to experience.[2]

When the session started, much to my surprise my practitioner gave more attention to my belly than to my outturned right leg. She spent a great deal of time softly holding and gently rocking my belly. Later she told me it felt as if I had a frightened child within my hard coconut shell of a belly, and it needed reassurance. "If you don't feel safe, you won't let me in, and then you'll never get the feeling you're searching for."

For homework she instructed me to say hi to my belly and gently paint smiles on it with my hands, not expecting anything, not judging anything, just feeling the sensation. Two or three sessions and a lot of homework later, my practitioner, through her gentle movements and mindful connection, reintroduced into my body/mind what it would *feel* like to have a belly that was soft, peaceful, and light.

After that I melted to her touch. Both consciously and unconsciously, I trusted. I automatically opened to receive new feelings. This time, she focused on my right leg, rolling it to the center again and again to give me a feeling of how it could be if it were straight. For homework, she gave me Mentastics, or mental gymnastics, to practice. She taught me to imagine a dinosaur tail extending off my tailbone for tripod-like stability. In the days to come, I practiced straightening my right foot and sitting on my tail whenever I noticed myself in my compensating stance.

Soon my trust grew deeper, and the feeling of a safe belly grew stronger. Using baby steps at first, I let go of the anxiety in my belly while learning what it felt like to stand in my center with a straight right leg.

I had caught the feeling from this practitioner. In Hook-Up she laid her hands on my body and transferred into my unconscious as much of the feeling of the Life Force as I felt safe to allow. This feeling gave me other options to choose from. Suddenly the affirmation that I was exploring the strength of my center had effect.

No longer did I have to find my balance by skewing my right leg. I stood taller and held my head higher. The dysfunctional beliefs regarding my ability to stay balanced in a crisis, which I'd thought were a permanent part of my makeup, started to evaporate. For the first time in my life I could safely stand with balance and softness and just be who I was, in the moment, feeling peace.

This was just one step of many I would take to clear my body/mind of its impediments and blockages to the Life Force. And, to tell the truth, this process has never stopped, because I have continued to grow and experience life. We are all like an onion that has to be peeled — we remove one layer, and then another and another, wondering if we will ever get to the center... until at last we realize we *are* the center, emerging and expanding.

CHAPTER SIX

But What If I Can't Feel?

Come and be with me.
I will not know your arrival, but still come.
My mind will be too busy to notice your presence,
But please . . . come.
Sit with me at my foundation.
Make space for yourself amongst my crowded relics.
Your help is requested.
Bring your hammer and chisel.
Together we will change
The parameters of my existence.
Vaguely, I will be aware of a shift.
At first it will seem ever so slight,
But I know the reverberations
Will rock my mind
And change my life.

— PAUL LATOUR

Many of us have been taught to ignore or discount our feelings and therefore are unable to consciously *feel* the results of the Life Force running through our bodies. Axioms such as "Big boys don't cry" and "Professionals don't bring emotion to the business table" push our wealth of intelligent feelings behind a self-erected wall. *Out of sight, out of mind*, we think, convincing ourselves we are devoid of feelings — or at least that we have none worth investigating, let alone listening to.

People who treat feelings this way (and in my younger days I fell into this category) convince themselves that the body is merely a vehicle to carry around the brain and that the brain is merely a vehicle for the mind. I have a dear friend, a spiritual buddy of thirty years, who believes this. When we get together (which isn't as often as I'd like), we invariably get into a discussion of our different points of view. The last time was over a glass of wine in his book-cluttered living room.

"You have to include the body in the enlightenment package," I said. "Through the body and the feelings it has, we interact with and interpret the field of energy that is the Unified Field. You know, that place we're all longing to get to."

He placed his wineglass on the sand-filled hourglass end table and leaned forward — as if he were ready for a mock battle. "Not necessarily," he said with a good-natured raise of his eyebrow. "It's the mind that houses our consciousness. It's the mind that becomes enlightened. The body is just an illusion."

"No, no, no," I countered passionately. "The body is a manifestation of our consciousness. It's here for us to anchor our experiences and give us unbiased feedback regarding our beliefs and holding patterns, which are" — I leaned forward to emphasize my point — "the very things that hold back bliss from flowing into us right here, right now!"

He sat up straight, his breath leaving his body in a slow exhalation. "I beg to differ," he said with reserve. "The only use of the body is to house the mind. What happens to the body is of no other consequence. You cannot attain perfect enlightenment until you let go of the body. It is the heaviest, grossest manifestation of creation — full of flaws, the last remains of ignorance."

"But the flaws are doing their best to tell you something. Why do you think your neck always hurts?"

"My neck isn't telling me anything. My spine pops out of alignment, which causes my neck to get sore. It's purely a mechanical problem. End of story. You're putting too much meaning on what happens in the body."

"Well, it's been my experience that a purely mechanical problem is a message, a physical manifestation of some belief or habitual way of being that is holding you back from the very thing you want most. It's saying to you, 'Look at me! Look at me! I am your way to nirvana!'"

My friend just shook his head. "Sometimes, my dear," he said, "a cigar is just a cigar!"

At this point in such a conversation, I usually throw up my hands in resignation and laughingly agree to disagree.

I love this old friend dearly, but I sometimes wonder if he is acting like an ostrich, burying his head in the hope that if he ignores his discomfort it will go away. And for his sake, and the sake of many others, I hope it does. Unfortunately, as a Trager practitioner of several decades, it has been my experience that it does not.

❈

I had another friend who was in a bad relationship. Her mate was always flirting with other women. Instead of telling him that his behavior hurt her, she made excuses for him. "He can't help it. He's so good-looking, women just come on to him."

Over and over her self-esteem was ground to dust as she witnessed his behavior. I asked her once, "Why don't you talk to him, tell him how you feel about having to witness this so often?"

She shifted her eyes to the ground, "Oh, it's really not that bad; I'm just venting. And, anyway, I hate confrontations."

"But won't you feel better if you deal with the issue?"

"I'm fine, really I am."

"Have you at least talked to him about it?"

She again looked away. "Well, I tried once but he said he didn't know what I was talking about, so I let it go. It's my problem if I feel uncomfortable; it means I don't trust him."

"Didn't you tell me a month or so ago that you were developing heartburn and thought you might have an ulcer?"

She waved her hand in a dismissive gesture, "Oh, my heartburn has nothing to do with him!"

I looked her in the eye. "Are you so sure?"

Trusting Our Bodies

Recurring backaches, continually stiff shoulders, persistent nauseated stomachs, or chronic headaches are not just the negative consequences of outside stresses. These symptoms and many others are also the body's way of reflecting back to us the quality of our labels and beliefs, and the way their subsequent holding patterns skew and distort the Life Force.

The body is trustworthy. Its responses are always authentic, never clouded by ego or self-delusion. We can trust the body. It too is intelligent. Discomfort and pain are messages, red flags to bring our attention to the E-motional patterns that lie at their root.

So heed your pain. It is a good thing. It can act as a reminder to come into presence and allow Spirit to clarify the message. The difficulty, however, is that many of us have blocked off any such communication as a survival mechanism against abuse. In whatever form, sexual, physical, or emotional abuse causes the unconscious to automatically create chemical changes that form an energetic wall, a kind of armor around the affected areas, which shuts them down — like going into shock. This action protects us against collapse, which is a good thing.

Only this armor stays. It doesn't dissipate. Years and decades later our automatic pilot has held the course. Protecting us, yes, but also disconnecting us from our source. Is it any wonder many of us can't feel or communicate with our unconscious?

Heavily armored people are not always obvious. They do not walk around like automatons. They still get angry, cry at funerals, and love their partner and children. But privately their feelings lack the depth and richness they are capable of achieving. They feel the reaction to situations but not the origin of the feeling. They are desperate for control. Desperate to keep their pain and discomfort contained.

To such people I would say: You don't have to jump off a cliff. You don't have to take a huge leap of faith. Simply foster a little willingness that perhaps there is something more. Open your mind to explore what might be. In my practice I have known many such people who, at first, had no physical experience of what I was talking about. With a little willingness, they have expanded their horizons and discovered that many of the things they thought were permanent tenants of their minds and bodies are not.

We have the free will and the creative ability to choose differently. If we don't like what's happening in our lives, as was the case with my turned-out right leg and subsequent unbalanced nature, we can make changes. We don't have to wait until our heartburn or tight neck or hard belly manifests into a greater trauma — a bigger wake-up call. We can learn to use our feelings as a way to communicate through our unconscious body/mind with Spirit.

CHAPTER SEVEN

Opening to the Life Force
A SAMPLE SESSION

N ow that we have touched upon the elements of our unconscious body/mind that can skew and impede the
flow of the Life Force, let's delve deeper into what happens in
actual Trager sessions. Let's discover *how* the Trager Approach
can bring us to a deeper place of feeling and connection, even
if we are at first out of touch with our unconscious patterning.

A determined, cherub-faced, postmenopausal woman
stepped into my treatment room and sat on the chair next to
my Trager table. During the pre-session interview, she talked
briefly about her history of sexual abuse. She told me how she
longed to be free of the nightmares and emotional handicaps
that kept her a victim, and ended by saying, "I can't cope
with anything. I have no energy, and every virus that comes
along attacks me. And nothing touches my heart, not love,
not even anger. I'm numb, a robot."

"Such reactions to trauma are not unusual," I said. "It's
only you taking care of yourself."

"Well, if I am, those strategies no longer work; I'm tired of being an empty shell."

"That's the autopilot of your unconscious doing its job," I assured her. "The traumas in your childhood probably caused your feelings to flee the scene as a protective mechanism. Your unconscious then put armor around your emotional body and set the dial to automatic. Trager can help you reset that dial and give your body other, more pleasurable feeling experiences to choose from."

My client ran her hands through her curly gray hair, leaned closer, and asked, "How can Trager take me out of this place? The friend who recommended you told me a little about what you do, but I don't really know how it works."

"Well," I said, "during a Trager session the practitioner — me in this instance — Hooks-Up or makes a connection with the Life Force, that unbounded reservoir of energy all around us, and then transfers the feeling experience of this connection to your body/mind through movement and touch. In this way you experience what it *feels* like to go beyond your fixed boundaries. It's like the measles — you catch it from someone who already has it. If you like the experience and find it safe enough, your unconscious mind will choose to drop its old pattern because the unconscious will always move toward what is more pleasurable. Letting go of such restrictions, stepping beyond your current boundaries, gives you a bigger playing field. And from this vaster place you have more choices. You can choose a different way to be, keep a more pleasurable feeling state, heal past wounds, live in the here and now. The more you open to this process, the deeper we will go."

"Sounds too good to be true. Can all that happen in one session?"

"It's possible," I said, "but usually a series of sessions is required. You, the client, at least the unconscious part of you, are in control. The release of old patterns occurs only when *you* feel safe enough to do so. Many people think they're willing, but if they look deeper inside they often find that they're not really; they are afraid it might bring up old stuff they don't want to revisit."

"Will it?" she asked. "Because a part of me is hesitant to reexperience the past. I don't want to feel that stuff ever again."

"I can't guarantee that you won't experience some of those old feelings," I told her. "But if you do, it will be akin to cleaning the muck out of your emotional pipes. Those old feelings will be leaving you rather than you taking them on again. We're not going to analyze your past. Trager doesn't work like that. That's the beauty of it. It doesn't erase your memories; it simply gives your body/mind another feeling experience to choose from in the here and now, and therefore the possibility of another way of being. It does this by going underneath the old patterns, straight to your foundation, where the energy of bliss, of peace, of light flows pure and unfettered. Does that sound like something you want to do?"

"I think so . . . yes, I do."

"Then, let's begin this process by exploring what is actually happening inside your body right now."

And I stood to lead her in the exploration of her own body movement using a few simple Mentastics. Soon she was shifting her weight from side to side, her long denim skirt swishing against the carpet as she played with gravity to find her center and become present. As she swayed, I asked her to scan her body and report what she noticed.

"I get pain when I move my hips to the right side," she said. "It feels stuck."

"Then pull the movement back until there's no pain, even if you have to reduce the movement to only a thought in your mind. Pushing through resistance only produces more opposition. In Trager we always do less when encountering resistance. This allows that area of your body/mind to feel safe and therefore let go."

Her eyes closed. Her movement slowed, then stopped altogether. She took a slow luxurious in-breath, and on the exhalation a subtle but leisurely movement flowed from her hips like the gentle sway of kelp in the ocean.

After a few moments I asked her to bring her movements to a close, then suggested she stand on a short stool with her right foot dangling over the side. "Now drop your hip and playfully rotate your leg while keeping your ankle and knee soft." As she did so I instructed her to ask her leg, "What could be freer?" and to notice if she felt a shift.

She giggled in embarrassment at my seemingly childish request. So I told her she didn't need to ask out loud; she could do it in her mind. Very soon I noticed a soft bounce in her tissue and promised her (because she was unable to detect this shift) that the process was beginning to work already.

Afterward, I brought these initial Mentastics to a close and instructed her on the next phase of her treatment — table work. "Take off as much or as little clothing as you feel comfortable with and then lie face up on the table, under the blanket."

Her shoulders dropped as if some weight had been taken off.

"Trager works well through clothing," I assured her. "We don't use oils or lotions, so there is no need to undress if it is uncomfortable for you. And leave your underpants on regardless. I'll be rocking and jiggling your tissue in order to transfer the feeling of Hook-Up into the deepest core of your bones and nervous system, so clothing makes no difference."

I left the room to wash my hands and allow her time to get ready. When I returned I started the table session by bringing *myself* into the present moment. I adopted the innocence of Beginner's Mind, then performed my own Mentastics. I focused on the ground beneath my feet. I sat on my imaginary tail and raised my arms — palms up — to feel the weight of my hands. I lengthened my diaphragm by adding a skyhook (the imaginary hook at the crown of my head that pulled me toward the heavens) and breathed into my full chest.

Ah, yes — that feeling!

Hooked-Up to the Life Force, I started at my client's head and neck. With soft, velvety hands I lightly invited her to experience the weight of her head as I rhythmically moved her neck. The soothing, nonintrusive movement soon lulled her into a relaxed and open state. I asked within, *What could be lighter?* and her neck let go even more.

Next I moved to her legs and feet. As I explored her right leg, I noticed that one of her strongest holding patterns was in the adductor muscles of her thigh. When I invited her leg to open, the adductor muscle (which squeezes the thighs together) resisted; she didn't want to let me open her leg. So I rocked, elongated, jiggled, and fluffed her leg to show her unconscious mind what it felt like to have a leg free from restriction. As I noticed her tissue letting go and softening, I anchored the feeling by saying, "There, that feeling. Did you notice that?"

"No, I didn't feel anything. Will I ever be normal?"

"Of course you will," I said. "We'll just take it one small step at a time. The safer you feel, the more you will let go."

As I continued to explore her leg while in Hook-Up, I asked her to close her eyes and say hello to her leg, thus strengthening the communication we had started earlier with Mentastics between her conscious body/mind, her unconscious body/mind, and the Life Force. Next, I suggested that she ask her leg, "What could feel softer?" and that she acknowledge the response when she felt a shift.

"I still can't feel anything!"

"It's okay; you will," I said. I continued to imprint each shift by saying, "Yes, that feeling," when I noticed her tissue respond.

Even though she could not consciously feel the shifts occurring in her tissue, the memory of this feeling experience was now stored in her unconscious — her database. After the session, as homework, I gave her more Mentastics to practice in order to anchor what her body/mind had learned from the session. Along with the movement explorations, I told her to ask herself, "What did it feel like when I was on the table?" This recall exercise would pave the way to a clearer interpretation and experience of the Life Force.

During the next session, as I explored her right leg again, I noticed the adductor muscles continued to hold resistance: She still did not want to let me open her leg. In response, I gently laid it down and stepped back from the table. I needed to move even more profoundly into presence, to go deeper in my communication with her holding pattern — but even lighter, even less threatening with my touch. I paused, took a deep breath. I felt my feet and my earth connection through my imaginary tail, my length and lightness through my sky-hook. I felt the weight of my upturned palms and readopted the innocent explorer attitude of Beginner's Mind, reinforcing the present moment within myself and deepening my connection to the Life Force. I now had greater access to the Unified Field, to that transcendental art store that supplies infinitely versatile material of the purest quality.

I stepped to the table again and started ever so lightly to rock her leg, transferring this feeling of profound connection. We were Hooked-Up to the flow, beyond her holding pattern, past her dysfunction, to the source of all possibilities. I stayed receptive, open with intention, allowing the energy of the Life Force to flood her leg.

This time she felt safe enough to trust. She was at a choice point. Her unconscious chose to accept this new feeling. She let go. I felt a melting sensation in her tissue. Then screams, tears, and gestures erupted — her unconscious had chosen to express what had been frozen in time. Her leg kicked out with each scream.

Over and over.

After a while, her sobs and kicking subsided, and she was able to dry her tears, blow her nose, and take a series of deep, cleansing breaths. She agreed to carry on. When I began to work on the back of her right leg, it continued to play out the drama by silently kicking until it finished releasing the bound energy of the holding pattern.

After the session, she paused on her side for a few moments to give her body/mind time to process the experience. "You know," she confessed, "it was my right side that was always facing the edge of the bed. He always touched my right leg first." And she gave a last shudder.

When she was ready I helped her to her feet. "Let's integrate these new boundaries into your feeling database," I said. "Let's do a few Mentastics. Feel the bottoms of your feet and sit on your tail — it can be any kind of tail you want as long as it trails on the ground. Pause with that feeling.... Good. Now, imagine a skyhook attached to the top of your head, going into the heavens. Feel the length in your diaphragm. As you breathe, open and close your chest like an umbrella...wonderful. Now, shift your weight as we did at the beginning of the session...fantastic. Bring your attention to your hips. How do they feel now?"

"Much lighter," she said, softly swaying like kelp again. "Fabulous. And I can move them all the way over to the right — effortlessly, as if you've poured warm oil in all my joints."

"This is how it feels to operate from your source," I said. "Take the time to let your body/mind register the experience. Just feeling the shift of weight will keep you in the present moment, and you can do *that* anytime, anywhere."

"I feel so grounded and secure somehow, yet I want to go running and jumping and playing on the beach. Maybe I'll go build a sand castle!"

"Sounds great," I said. "Just be gentle with yourself for at least twenty-four hours to allow everything to settle into its new form. I would suggest a warm bath or a nice walk — something playful but light."

"You're right. I don't want to go blasting through some of the more delicate feelings. I guess I'll take my time to explore my new hips."

"When you're practicing Mentastics, remember to ask, 'How did my hips feel after the session?' It will activate a positive feedback response."

"I will. And thank you."

❈

Because I connected with this woman *beyond* the trauma of her sexual abuse, she experienced freedom as a feeling in her leg. The release of this holding pattern didn't mean the memory of her experience was erased — no one can erase negative memories; they are forever stored in our unconscious. Instead, with the Trager Approach, she experienced the Life Force while in the present moment, which brought with it, through her unconscious, a new choice into her awareness.

CHAPTER EIGHT

Releasing Holding Patterns

Keeping the connection to our source all of the time, in every situation, requires us to get reacquainted with the present moment. Trager teaches us kinesthetically (in a body-movement experience) how to do this. It also helps clear any impediments in our unconscious that keep us from the here and now.

In Trager, as we learned earlier, we call these impediments to the Life Force *holding patterns*. They, along with our labels and beliefs, distort the feelings of lightness, bliss, and peace continuously coming to us from the Unified Field.

Think of holding patterns as blocks of ice in the mind, holding rigid an otherwise free-flowing way of being in the world. If the mind holds some rigidity, that rigidity naturally spills into the body and we experience blocks, tightness, and perhaps pain and illness. Our posture reflects this inflexibility as our unconscious forms a pattern in order to cope. For example, if we believe that to open our hearts to another will only bring hurt, then this is often reflected in the shoulders, upper chest, and neck as stiffness, compression, and pain, because we may be unconsciously "holding" the heart together. This holding pattern is like a dam of icebergs impeding the flow of an otherwise free-moving body of water. Water that isn't allowed to move becomes stagnant, bringing disruption and *dis-ease* — in this case perhaps chronic bronchitis, asthma, heart disease, or any number of other maladies associated with the chest and heart.

When we start playing around in the present moment, inviting the energy of the Life Force into our conscious life, these old patterns start to unwind and release from our body/mind. When the ice melts we actually feel our energy coming from a deeper, more stable source. We feel more awake, more present, lighter.

These releases are best expected and welcomed. They can happen all at once or gradually through a series of sessions that "melt the ice." I would love to tell you that the process of releasing these old holding patterns — these stiff backs, tight shoulders, hard bellies, and chronic headaches — will always be wonderful and blissful, but unfortunately I cannot. Sometimes the shift is gentle and pleasurable and sometimes it is painful and volatile. I can promise you, however, that as the process unfolds you *will* feel lighter and more expansive, and you *will* automatically move toward more empowerment and a fuller, richer life. In other words, it's worth it. I've seen it time and again. I've experienced it for myself.

The Process of Release

Do not go where the path may lead,
Go instead where there is no path
And leave a trail.

— RALPH WALDO EMERSON

Let's take another look at the process of release, so you will have some idea of what to expect. Again, imagine the body/mind as a large pipe or conduit that has been clogged with the mud and debris from the overload of our life experiences. Connecting to the present moment is akin to opening a valve that sends pure clean water (the energy of the Life Force) through the pipe. Each time it courses through, it cleans out a little more of the muck that has impeded the flow. How we feel as this debris is released depends on what clogged the pipe in the first place. For example, in the last chapter we saw that if the trauma of sexual abuse has been clogging the pipe, the release might be tears and screams and violent movement. But if the clog has formed from a repetitive motion due to too much work, the release might be a deep sense of softness and relief.

As our pipes clear, we release the clogged energy that has been bound to us through a dysfunctional belief and its physical counterpart, a holding somewhere in the body. In a Trager session when the client is ready to open to the Life Force in a deeper way, the practitioner experiences a softening of the tissue and an overall feeling of lightness and ease. The client experiences a sensation much like being heard for the first time, which causes the client to feel safe and therefore let go. This allows the Life Force to flow through the body/mind, expelling some of the muck. Such a release may be expressed as a deep cleansing breath, a yawn, a gurgle in the belly, a sniff or cough, cries, laughter, spasms, shouts — the list goes on and on. Afterward, the client often feels expansive, light, and delicious. But not always. Sometimes a release takes longer, especially if it is a deep-seated holding pattern, which is why after a session I tell clients to be gentle with themselves for at least twenty-four hours as their systems realign. Once this realignment is complete, lightness comes and more choices arrive.

Mentastics can help us during those challenging times. They can be used as a regulating tool so we are not at the mercy of E-motions unwinding from their holding patterns. We can learn to ground the awareness of the Life Force by becoming present through Hook-Up as we move through our days. In this way, we anchor this connection in our body/mind, which smoothes out the release process.

❧

Do you remember when, during my Level 1 Trager Professional Training, I burst into tears in front of all those people I barely knew, believing myself to be inadequate because I wasn't learning as quickly as my inner perfectionist figured I should? That was a release of expectation around who I *thought* I should be.

During this episode of letting go, the instructor helped me to feel safe and adequate, explaining that it was okay not to get it right off, that we all have our own learning curve and style. Then afterward she led me through some Mentastics — thereby connecting me to the Life Force, which helped to ease and regulate the release process. She instructed me to feel my feet, to sit on my tail, to breathe into my umbrella, and ask myself, *What could be easier?*

The kinesthetic response I received anchored me and kept me from identifying with either the releasing process or my old dysfunctional belief that I had to learn quickly and perfectly the first time around. "Remember," my instructor said, "it is just energy moving through your system. What does unfettered flow feel like?"

For the entire second half of the training week, I allowed myself to become steeped in the idea of Beginner's Mind, and to some degree stayed in a constant state of Hook-Up. I touched others — and was touched and moved by others — more during that week than in my entire life's experience up to that date. I absorbed the purity found in the Life Force through this special touch.

When I got home, I seemed to dance effortlessly through space with every gesture. For days I could almost see the sparkle of my wake as I moved my arm through the air. I felt as if I had been taken to the top of a mountain and shown the magnificent 360-degree view — I had a bigger playing field. Wow!

For the following week this feeling of expansiveness stayed, but then it faded as my old ways of being reasserted themselves. It was like being taken back down to the base of the mountain, where my task was to cut a path of my own to the top, while in the process overturning every rock and smelling every flower along the way.

I would need to remind myself many times before my new habits had a strong hold. I had to commit to the intention of having this pure experience on a regular basis. I had to commit to doing Mentastics — to pause, to breathe into my umbrella, to feel my weight, to ask what could be more effortless, especially when I was feeling rushed or overwhelmed.

Practicing Mentastics helped to smooth out any psychological and physiological complaints my old dysfunction belted out. This, combined with receiving Trager sessions whenever possible, anchored my awareness of the Life Force in my everyday waking life. Over time, because of my deepened connection, my unconscious body/mind automatically and effortlessly chose confidence over fear and empowerment over inadequacy, all within an envelope of safety.

And yours can too.

More on Mentastics

The Mentastics in this book have been designed to bring the present moment into conscious awareness. Some only require you to be mentally active (Mentastics 2, for example), while others require movement to get the feeling. If the instructions suggest movement but you are physically challenged and cannot stand, then sit. If you cannot sit, remain lying down. Have the intention of starting each part of the Mentastics in your imagination; then bring the movement as far into the body as you can. For instance, if you cannot stand to shift weight with your feet, feel the bottoms of your feet and shift the weight of your bottom on a chair. If you are lying down, roll your head from side to side, or imagine yourself standing and shifting your weight from side to side.

Mentastics 3:
Regulating the Release of a Holding Pattern

1. Stand easily with your feet shoulder-width apart. (Sit or lie comfortably if you cannot stand.) Pause a moment. . . . Breathe into your belly, diaphragm, and chest as if you were opening an umbrella. . . . Bring your awareness to the bottoms of your feet (to help, you can picture them or wiggle your toes).

2. Close your eyes. Slowly shift your weight from side to side. Scan your body with your mind, and find a part where you would like to feel a change. Maybe the area feels stiff or painful or restricted in some way.

3. Continue to shift your weight slowly from side to side. Notice as you move what happens to that area. How does it feel?

4. Now, as you shift, ask the area, *What could feel softer?* and wait with Beginner's Mind for the answer to come. (Does it come as a thought, a feeling, a picture?) Pause. . . . Breathe into the area. . . . Notice how it feels.

5. Shift your weight again. Notice how it feels now.

6. Ask, *What could be softer than that?* and wait with innocence for the answer to come. Pause. . . . Breathe into the area.

7. Continue to shift your weight slowly, still focusing on the same area. Ask, *How can this softness go deeper inside?* Wait with Beginner's

Mind for the answer to come. Pause.... Breathe into the area.... Notice.

8. Shift your weight yet again and again notice the feeling. Ask, *And can this softness go deeper than that?* With innocence wait for the answer. Pause.... Breathe into the area.

9. Continue this questioning process until you experience some release, then...Pause.... Breathe.... Notice the new feeling.

10. Breathe into this feeling to own it.

Releasing holding patterns can be a beautiful or challenging experience. We can view this letting-go process as a positive cleansing or just one more negative aspect of life we have to bear. Our choice will influence the atmosphere around which the holding pattern unfolds. In order to have a positive experience, we need not push away our anger, pain, or anxiety. Staying with the energy while grounded in the Life Force allows it to fully unwind. Not judging our sensations and subsequent releases as good or bad but instead realizing that we are just letting go of the results of our overloads allows for a smoother transition into a new way of being.

INTERLUDE ONE

I n part I we were introduced to lots of information, so let's
take a couple of pages to recap what we learned. We learned
that our feelings (like electromagnets) are the true power in
our life, attracting to us situations and relationships that mirror the colors of our emotions. We learned that when we
Hook-Up to the life-giving, life-regulating power that is all
around us, we experience feelings of peace, of bliss, of light
— feelings that in turn change the dynamics of our inner life
and then our outer life.

This power we Hook-Up to is the Life Force, the active
expression of the Unified Field, our source, the starting
point, the place where everything is one and the same. The
Life Force is nonlinear and nonlocal, but most important it
is intelligent. And if we are willing it will guide us (infinitely
better than our intellectual ego-self) along lines of least resistance toward a transformation into who our Spirit wants us
to become.

Remember, if we were to paint a linear picture of how the Life Force flows, it would look something like this:

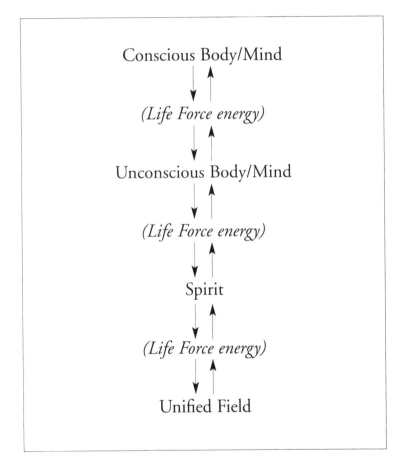

Conscious Body/Mind

(Life Force energy)

Unconscious Body/Mind

(Life Force energy)

Spirit

(Life Force energy)

Unified Field

We have also learned that the dynamics of our unconscious body/mind are, to a large extent, responsible for the quality of our feelings and therefore the direction of our life. This is because our unconscious functions as transmitter, translator, and filter between our conscious body/mind and our Spirit. Through our unconscious the energy of the Life Force (E-motion, energy in motion) is channeled.

Unfortunately, impediments or blockages in our unconscious body/mind can radically skew our interpretation and partially block the bliss, the peace, the light coming through Spirit. For this reason it is important to become conscious of the interconnected web of components operating within our unconscious. These components are labels, beliefs, and their corresponding holding patterns. Again, labels are definitions we give to particular energy patterns in our bodies. Associating one or more of these labels with a certain situation over time causes a belief to form. Holding patterns and their resultant postures are the psychological and physical mirrors of our beliefs. Together, these components form a web that either holds us back or propels us forward.

Moreover, we have discussed the idea of Beginner's Mind and why it is important to adopt a state of innocence in which each moment is fresh, clear, and open. By giving ourselves permission to *not* know, *not* expect, and *not* compare, we open up our usual narrow perception and unburden ourselves from comparisons, past mistakes, and future expectations. With Beginner's Mind, our feelings become our compass. By minding our feelings we can choose actions and attitudes that elicit bliss over guilt, peace over turmoil, love over fear, and forgiveness over resentment.

We have also journeyed through an in-depth Trager session and seen how a practitioner can transfer into a client's tissue the feeling experience of what it would be like without outdated holding patterns and beliefs, using Mentastics to further reeducate our nervous system.

In addition, we have discussed the possible ramifications of the release of old holding patterns that have been gumming up the conduit of our body/mind.

At every step along the way, the one point we have kept circling back to is the present moment. In the present moment we automatically Hook-Up to the Life Force, giving us more lightness, more bliss, more peace. In the present moment our empowerment, our clarity, our creativity, and our long-term productivity automatically increase. In the present moment contentment and passion arise naturally and effortlessly. In the present moment we find Spirit.

Arriving into the present moment is the bottom line of the Trager Approach, and it is what part 2 of this book will focus on. Dr. Milton Trager developed a whole range of tools to help practitioners enter the present moment. We will look at just six of these because, from my experience, they are the easiest for a non-Trager practitioner to use, and serendipitously they are the most fundamental. These six tools are:

1. Pausing
2. Mindful umbrella breathing
3. Feeling the weight
4. Questioning
5. Trusting ourselves not to know
6. Finding our rhythm

PART TWO

TOOLS TO GET THERE

I said to the wanting-creature inside me:
What is this river you want to cross?
There are no travellers on the road, and no road.
Do you see anyone moving about on that bank, or resting?
There is no river at all, no boat, and no boatman.
There is no towrope either, and no one to pull it.
There is no ground, no sky, no time, no bank, no ford!

And there is no body, and no mind!
Do you believe there is some place that will make the soul less thirsty?
In that great absence you will find nothing.

Be strong then, and enter into your own body:
There you will have a solid place for your feet.
Think about it carefully!
Don't go off somewhere else!

Kabir says this: just throw away all thoughts of imaginary things,
And stand firm in that which you are.

— KABIR (TRANSLATED BY ROBERT BLY)

CHAPTER NINE

Pause...Breathe...
Feel the Weight

There is no hurry,
There is no race,
I allow myself to move,
at a gentler pace.

Of haste and hurry,
I have no need,
All will be well,
If I pause and breathe.

— SUSAN HEALEY

On the one hand we may say we want to arrive in the present moment and welcome the unfettered Life Force into our conscious life, while on the other hand most of us are resistant. Despite wanting to keep that Hook-Up feeling as we drive to work, make love to a partner, feed our kids, make our beds, dig in our gardens, we can't (for the most part) actually do it. We balk at the starting gate, spinning our wheels in frustration (which some call procrastination). Why? Because of fear. We are afraid of what we will become when we get rid of all the garbage that has clogged the conduit of our body/mind, shackling our life. We are afraid (consciously or unconsciously) to let go of our beliefs and the holding patterns they create. We are afraid to let go of an intimate friend.

Old patterns are like old friends who are comforting in their familiarity, even if we pay a price for the friendship. Discarding an old friend, a familiar way of being, a bad habit, or a repetitive action can be a fearful experience. If we choose to embrace the present moment, who would we become then? The more we experience the light, harmonious feelings inherent in the Unified Field, the more our life will change — that's guaranteed. To do so brings us into an unknown way of being, and it is this prospect of the unknown that threatens our old patterning and limiting beliefs.

The aspect of our consciousness that *identifies* with our "old friends" believes that if we allow ourselves to live in a new way there's a good chance it will be annihilated, gone from existence, wiped out like chalk from a chalkboard. From this perspective, it's a life-or-death struggle for that aspect of our consciousness to hold on to who it *thinks* we are. In effect we're asking this part of ourselves to put its identity, its very life, on the line. Is it any wonder we have built up a mountain of fear over change?

It is important to remind the part of ourselves that identifies with our old patterns that it will not be lost. The Life Force will not wash away our identity, merely our old, worn-out clothing. There is no way for us to lose ourselves by embracing the Life Force. In fact, the reverse is true; all that will happen is we will become more fully who we authentically are.

To further alleviate this fear, it is also important to keep the process of change practical and simple, yet flexible enough to synchronize with our unique rhythms. The six tools I mentioned in the interlude will do this. They will carve steps into our mountain of fear, giving us safe footholds. Each time we use these tools, they will safely and actively clear a path, aligning us more closely with the Life Force and our Spirit.

Pausing

The first tool is … pausing.

Before we can consciously open to the Life Force, we have to apply the breaks to our *doing*, both in our mind and body. We have to stop talking, stop walking, stop washing the dishes, stop worrying, fretting, controlling … and pause.

If we're driving a car full tilt down the road and we want to turn a corner, what do we do? Do we crank the wheel while still at top speed? No way — we'd skid out of control and end up a pile of rubble in the ditch. Similarly, fear of an emotional crash if we turn a corner keeps us traveling down the same old road. In response to our fear, the Trager Approach offers a safer way to begin a change. We gently apply the brakes, slow down, clear our mind … pause. When movement is slowed, we have the power to mindfully turn a corner.

A pause enables us to step out of our particular experience and listen to our inner feeling voice, the thread of our

Spirit connected to the Unified Field. A pause helps us to become the observer instead of the reactor. It is a gateway that opens onto a path that leads to empowerment. It is also the hardest step to take.

❧

I was at the base of the mountain. Looking up, I could only marvel at where I had been after my Level 1 Trager training only months earlier. My old patterns and habits had pushed out the effortless movement I had been given. I knew I needed to commit to using the tools I had learned. I knew my task was to cut a path of my own to the top, while overturning every rock and smelling every flower. I knew this, but it was as if the pendulum had swung back the other way; I was unable even to use the first tool I had learned — to pause.

I had to keep on top of things. I had to be productive. I had a household to run and two active, hungry boys to care for. So when I was vacuuming or cooking or doing the laundry and noticed a soreness in my right hip, I wouldn't stop. Just a couple of more minutes and I'll take a break, I'd promise myself, and I'd lean into my work even more. It was a bargain: First I'll finish the chore, and then I'll take the time for my hip. But when I was done, something else often got in the way: a neighbor dropping by, my sister calling, the boys bursting in wanting attention....

Although I wanted to cease my old ways, I didn't have the power to take the first step. Intellectually I wanted to reexperience the wonder and bliss of my Level 1 training, but parts of me were afraid to let go of what they knew. My familiar friends — those old patterns and limiting beliefs — had built up momentum in my life, making it difficult not to identify with them.

When I'd reflect upon my procrastination, I could only remind those parts of my consciousness that my identity would not be annihilated, simply given a new set of clothes. By going lighter instead of plowing through, I affirmed my intent to change without giving my dysfunction a wall to push back against.

This cycle of bargaining and reassuring continued for several months before I finally was able to slow down the speeding car of my body/mind. It happened late afternoon on New Year's Eve. I was preparing for the family celebration my husband, sons, and I had planned. I had vacuumed and dusted the house, and cleaned the bathrooms. I had just put the rugs back on the polished kitchen floor and was taking vegetables out of the fridge to cut up and put out as part of our feast when my right hip started to ache. Worried because it was getting late and I still had to set the dining room table after I finished preparing the food, I stepped up the pace. The ache in my hip escalated to a burn. It was trying to tell me something. I bargained as usual. *Just let me finish these preparations, and then I'll stop and have a soak in the tub.* A streak of white-hot lightning shot up my back.

Slow down! I could practically hear my right hip shout. This time I could no longer ignore the message.

"Okay, okay. I'll stop," I yelled out loud.

I stepped away from the cutting board and, with a groan, placed my hands on my lower back, put the brakes on my motoring mind, and...paused. I felt the soft rug under my feet. A swell of that same softness flooded up my legs and over my hips. My pelvis sighed. The sensation wasn't much, but enough to remind my hip what it felt like when I was Hooked-Up during my Level 1 training. I played with this feeling for a moment until I noticed it seep into my mind. My thinking softened effortlessly: *So what if I'm not finished before everyone comes back from tobogganing. I'll just recruit them to help with the setup; that way they will feel more involved.* As it turned out I was able to finish with ease, leaving the decorating of the side table to them.

My procrastinating took months; pausing took about thirty seconds!

⚜

With my pause I took another step. I committed. It was the first time since I returned home from my training that I consciously chose to listen to my body — if only when it was screaming. By utilizing this initial tool, I slowed down the speeding car of my mind, putting some distance between my "shoulds" and me. It was this initial break away from my conditioning, my patterned way of being, that was so difficult.

Let's take a moment to do a little Mentastics. I know you probably want to rush on to the next tool, to the rest of the information, to the goal of finishing this book, but instead, stop.

Apply the breaks.

Slow down.

Pause....

Mentastics 4: Pausing

1. Get comfortable....Breathe....Close your eyes for a count of three leisurely breaths.
2. Open your eyes, and breathe in again.... Great. You have experienced what a pause feels like. Easy, yes?
3. Now, let's take pausing into our actions. Sit comfortably upright in a solid chair. (For those who are not mobile, follow along in your mind or use the same principles for any part of your body that does move.)
4. Pause....Have the intention to rise from the chair....But before you do...pause....
5. Plant your feet solidly on the floor in front of you. Pause....
6. Stand up. Pause again....
7. Start walking around the room, noticing how your feet meet the floor. When you find you are not paying attention to how your feet meet the floor...pause....
8. Resume walking, paying attention to the bottoms of your feet. Each time your mind strays from noticing your feet...pause....

Congratulations. You've paused. You've succeeded in applying the most difficult tool. You've slowed your conditioning. You've reached a place of decreased momentum, of rest. The more you pause the more you will remember to pause, ushering in a whole new avenue of possibilities.

Mindful Umbrella Breathing

After pausing with intention, the next tool is . . . mindful umbrella breathing.

Out of all the processes that operate in our body, breathing is the one that connects us most strongly to Spirit. The act of breathing not only circulates atmospheric gases; it circulates the Life Force as well. When we focus on breathing our attention goes inside, to the conduit of our body/mind and the thread of our Spirit, where our center resides. From here it is easy to feel the flow of the Life Force.

Mindful umbrella breathing is the easiest of the tools to use, because when we pause, the body automatically takes a deep breath. When we pay attention to that breath (and hopefully subsequent ones as well), we become centered and therefore move toward an observer's perspective. It is like moving toward the hub of a wheel. Nearer to our hub, our perspective broadens, becoming multifaceted. Our assumptions soften, as does our identification with our emotions and their corresponding labels and beliefs. We realize we are not the pains we feel, or the thoughts we have — they are only one spoke of our wheel. We have stepped away from the rim, toward our center. From here we are able to observe more clearly what we are *actually* experiencing, rather than what we *think* we are experiencing.

Stepping away from the rim of the wheel does not mean jumping down an escape hatch as a way to hold ourselves back from living life fully, from loving and grieving fully, from laughing and crying fully. Being the observer doesn't mean that we stop caring; it simply takes us out of the place where we are overwhelmed by what is happening.

A ringing echoed along the gorge of my hallway, demanding to be answered. I marched to the door — *Can't people leave me alone?* — and threw it open. "Don't you understand? I don't want to see anyone!" I slammed the door shut. *Who was that?* I thought, about to storm away. *I can't remember.* Once more, the ringer blared. Wrenching the door wide, I shrieked, "Didn't you hear me? I want more breathing space!" I slammed the door shut again. But the ringing continued, over and over, until I surfaced out of my ocean of dreams.

I was in bed. It was six o'clock New Year's morning, and someone was calling — what nerve! And I had just fallen back to sleep after a bathroom visit. Why did my paranoia make me switch the phone back on?

Into the handset I croaked a froggy hello. I expected a cheery "Happy New Year!" Instead I got news that dropped the bottom out of my world.

Before that moment my world was white-picket-fence picture-perfect. With two kids, two cats, a new home, a husband with a good job, shares in a fledgling high-tech company, and a garden to play in, I had arrived. With so many reasons to be grateful, we had made the celebration of 1989 a memorable one. We had enjoyed a cheese fondue, followed by a chocolate one. There was sparkling juice and wine, party favors, card games, and Pink Floyd on the stereo. Jokes and laughter bubbled from the boys. And at midnight we'd hugged, toasted the New Year, and chorused "May old acquaintance be forgot. . . ." The party was for us, for our family. We'd wanted no interruptions. It was a conscious decision to turn off the phone.

Even so, throughout the evening I was nagged by a niggling sensation. *What if something happened? What if someone needed to get ahold of us? Shouldn't I be available? Shouldn't I take precautions?* Not wanting to dampen the festivities, I shoved these worries to the back of my mind, assuring myself that nothing could go wrong; I was just being paranoid.

When I picked up the receiver at six that morning, my earlier worries mocked me. My worst nightmare had come true. My sister-in-law had been calling all night. My stepfather was dead — my mother in shock.

Adrenaline surged through my body as I tried to absorb this blow. My face drained to a ghostlike mask. My mouth hung agape. A vise clamped around my chest. I couldn't breathe. The more I tried, the harder it became. My head became dizzy, my stomach nauseated. *Oh my God! Oh my God! I knew I shouldn't have turned off the phone. I knew it. How selfish to think I could shut out the world to suit myself. My mother, my mother! She needed me, and I wasn't there for her. I should have been. Oh God!*

My body crumpled. My mind grasped for a lifeline, something to grab onto. Then it came to me . . . pause.

I took no conscious action. The intent to pause was enough. It came to me; I did not go to it. My unconscious knew what I needed in that moment. My anxious thoughts drained like water down a sink. My chest softened. My lungs — *ffffffff* — emptied. My body unfurled as my lungs expanded in a much-needed deep, cleansing breath. Soon I could feel my chest, gently opening and closing like an umbrella.

With this initial reprieve, I remembered to imagine the air as energy rising from the center of the earth and flowing through my feet. I breathed into my vagina, my pubic bone, my belly, my chest, expanding my umbrella in a 360-degree circle. Then, slowly, with a soft exhalation, I sounded, "Ahh-hhhhh," as I imagined the trauma and pain of this horrific news leaving my body. I continued these Mentastics until I was no longer completely overwhelmed and had gained some perspective. Closer to the hub of my wheel now, I phoned the airlines, booked myself on the next flight, and threw what I needed into my worn blue suitcase.

❧

When we breathe with intention we aren't running away or ignoring feelings but rather finding balance. We are, after all, both the hub (the absolute) *and* the rim (the relative); we are called upon to encompass both. The ride of life often moves so fast out on the rim that it's hard to remember we are the hub as well. We identify with the rim, with the relative part of our existence, thereby creating a "this is me" feedback loop that keeps our beliefs and holding patterns rigid.

The act of pausing slows the spinning wheel. It breaks the momentum of our doing, both in mind and body, giving us a greater perspective and the opportunity to choose differently. And after the pause, the most natural gesture that creates an easy way to the absolute is mindful umbrella breathing. It extracts us from the world *out there* and connects us with the world *in here.*

Mentastics 5: Mindful Umbrella Breathing

1. Allow your body and mind to pause.... Take a slow in-breath. Breathe in the nourishing Life Force. Softly breathe out the oxygen-spent air.

2. While breathing in, imagine that you are bringing the Life Force up through the center of the earth, through imaginary golden roots attached to the bottoms of your feet. Breathe out any fatigue in your legs and feet.

3. Envision your next breath traveling up through your feet and flowing into your pubic bone, up to your belly and into your diaphragm. Again exhale, imagining yourself letting go of all your worries and judgments.

4. Breathe in once more, taking this life-giving energy all the way up into your chest, expanding your diaphragm and chest without arching your back or raising your shoulders. Exhale as you release all inadequacies, burdens, and strife.

5. Pause as you automatically breathe in through your roots once more. Notice how you feel.

6. With your next in-breath, imagine that your chest is an umbrella, with the point of the umbrella at the top of your head. Breathe in, opening the umbrella in a 360-degree circle; expand your front, back, and sides. Breathe out, closing the umbrella; expel toxin-filled, oxygen-spent air.

7. Breathe into your umbrella again. Feel this energy traveling up your torso, then along your arms and out your hands. Now slowly let the air out of your mouth, allowing all of the trauma, fatigue, and pain to leave your body in a sound ... ahhhhhh. Pause. ... Notice how you are feeling.

8. Bring your attention back to your breath. With your inner eyes, see the air traveling through your roots, into your legs, up your torso, and into your neck, spilling out the top of your head like a fountain of water. Pause. ... Notice how you are feeling.

9. Breathe into your umbrella again. Imagine this energy coming into the top of your head from above and sliding down your face and the back of your head onto your neck. Breathe out, and pause as you notice your out-breath tumbling down your body, soaking into the earth, being neutralized.

10. Breathe into your umbrella again and pause. ... Notice your feelings. Repeat as many times as necessary to reconnect with the hub of your wheel.

Feels good, doesn't it? Connecting to our source, to the Life Force, is a grounding, solidifying experience, and the more we have this experience, the more we will experience being centered, acting from a place of empowerment and grace. It's like that compounding interest account we talked about earlier.

Mindful umbrella breathing to find our source, however, is just one more part of the equation. To "have it all" we need to pay attention not only to the absolute world but to the relative world as well. We also need to be mindful of our physical bodies, of what is happening in the here and now. To do this, we use the third tool — feeling weight.

Feeling the Weight

Weight is the measure of the degree of downward pull produced by the earth's speed of rotation and gravitational field. The force of gravity attracts anything with mass (including our bodies) toward the center of the earth. Thinking the word *weight* can conjure up dense, sluggish sensations of heaviness. And yet, through attention to weight we can experience a lightness of being. This happens when the flow of the Life Force (which we have Hooked-Up to via our mindful umbrella breathing) is transferred into our tissue through feeling the weight of the body. By paying attention to the downward pull of gravity on a particular part — a hand, for example — as it moves through space, we cannot help but show up in the body, in the here and now. Feeling weight to become *lighter* works because the Life Force lives in the present moment; when we are Hooked-Up to it, it shares its characteristics of softness, lightness, and peace with us. I know this is a paradox. But try it. It works.

Every time we consciously feel the weight of our hands, or someone else's hand, or even a can of beans, we can put ourselves in the present moment. The next time you are putting the groceries away, doing the dishes, or lifting a hammer, feel the weight as you move the object through space. The next time you are holding the hand of someone you love, pause, breathe, and feel its weight. Allow yourself to give up its weight to gravity; rather than holding your loved one's hand up, let it rest in your palm. You will experience a noticeable difference. A positive life-affirming sensation will course through both of your bodies.

※

Twelve hours after that traumatic phone call, I walked into my mother's house and fell into the arms of my sister. Our skin, our hearts, and our minds seemed peeled away from shock and grief, and for a few moments we blended.

Through quiet tears, I whispered, "Where's Mom?"

"I put her on the couch," she whispered back and released me.

As I rounded the corner into the living room, my mother turned her blanched face and swollen red eyes to me. "I can't make it," she said in a thin, breathy voice. "I just can't. It's too much...I just can't..."

The grief was so big, what could I do? Death had never come to me in this way before. I could not know the extent of my mother's pain, so in that moment I did the only thing I could — I paused and breathed.

A thick fog of distress surrounded us. I pulled up a chair, sat down, and picked up her hand. "I know," I said. I closed my eyes for a minute, wanting so badly for my love to seep into her and give her strength. I slowly opened my eyes and, without a word, sat at her side with her hand in mine. Through the window behind the couch, a nearby branch of a cedar tree slowly bounced with the weight of January rains.

The movement echoed in my own hands as I began to feel the weight of my mother's hand. My chest expanded and contracted. My feet sank into the carpet, my bottom into the seat. I sat there, pausing, breathing, feeling myself be...on the chair...in the room...holding my mother's hand.

Soon, lightness seeped in, buoying my body and my heart. I noticed color creeping into my mother's face, her breath deepening with each rise and fall of her chest.

I Hooked-Up. My mother followed.

❧

By first pausing and breathing into our umbrellas, and then feeling weight, we open our bodies to the unbounded reservoir of the Unified Field. This can be done anytime, anywhere. While on a stroll, we can feel the weight of our arms as they swing. While waiting in line at the bank, we can shift our weight from side to side. While working on a keyboard, we can pay attention to the weight of our elbows hanging. Or, if discretion is in order, we can simply feel the weight of our jaw and the back of our neck. There is no time when we cannot feel the weight of some part of the body.

Mentastics 6: Feeling the Weight of Your Body

1. Allow your body and mind to pause....Breathe into your umbrella....Stand with your feet shoulder-width apart. Slowly and gently shift

your weight from one side to the other. Notice the shift of weight as it passes through the little bones in your feet. You are not here to judge, just to notice the sensations in your nervous system.

2. Now bring your attention to your ankles and notice the shift in weight. Pause, breathe, and notice...your calves...your knees.

3. Allow yourself to pause...and breathe.... Bring your awareness to your hips as they slowly shift from side to side. Feel the weight in the floor of your pelvis as it slides from side to side. Just notice.

4. Now bring your attention to your rib cage; feel the weight. Notice the feeling. Allow another pause.... Breathe.... Shift your weight from side to side, and bring your awareness to your shoulders. Notice how they feel.

5. Now down your arms and into your hands and fingers — feel the weight and notice.

6. Release your jaw, and feel its weight as you shift your body from side to side.

7. Feel the weight of your ears — first one and then the other. Allow yourself to pause... breathe...and notice.

8. Now expand your attention to encompass your whole body. How does your entire body shift as a unit? Take your time shifting side to side, and notice. Pause and breathe, and notice how you feel once more.

9. Now shift your weight backward and forward — just until your heels grab and just until your toes grab. Don't knock yourself off balance. Notice how the weight shifts differently from the way it did when you were going side to side.

10. Feel the weight in the front of your jaw and the back of your neck...in your chest and midback ...in your belly and low back...in the front of your thighs, in your quadriceps, and in the back of your thighs, your hamstrings....Pause and breathe....How do you feel? Light, I bet.

The tools of pausing to slow the momentum of our life, breathing to access our Spirit, and feeling weight to place our body and our mind in the present moment, bring together both the absolute and the relative, the spiritual and the physical. This is our place of personal power, the place where we can choose differently, less affected by our past conditioning or the changing tides of the fast-paced world around us. From here all the material from the transcendental art store (the Unified Field) is at our disposal.

❋

After the funeral did it get easier for me to stand in my place of power and choose these tools? Yes, though not immediately. I'd take the time to pause, breathe, and feel the weight one day, but not the next. My old friends — those outdated beliefs and corresponding holding patterns — would become convinced of their annihilation, grasping tightly to their tattered clothing. It took patience, reassurance, and willingness, but over time, with the help of these three simple tools, I made deepening inroads of trust with these friends. Together, my new resolve and my old identity discovered that the more we walked the path, the wider and clearer it became, making my connection to the Unified Field smoother and easier — and increasingly joyful.

Forming such a habit is akin to dipping a cloth in yellow dye. After immersing the cloth, we hang it outside to dry. As the sun beats down on it the color fades, so we dip it again in the dye, and again hang it in the sun. And again it fades. Over time the dye becomes fast. The dye is the Unified Field. The cloth is our body/mind. And the more we immerse ourselves in the experience of the Unified Field (found in the present moment), the more the feeling of it, the color of it, stabilizes in our nervous system.

All this can be realized by first pausing, then breathing and feeling weight.

CHAPTER TEN

Questioning

It is possible to dialogue with our unconscious. It's true: The parts of us above and below the waterline talk all the time, only they often don't understand one another. Few of us have been versed in the language of the unconscious.

How the Unconscious Communicates

Although the unconscious can use a dream, or an inner voice, or a private snapshot to speak to us, our body is its most consistent vehicle of communication. A soft, supple body flowing with blissful emotion says one thing; a body riddled with tension and pain says another. Because the unconscious body/mind is our filter and translation matrix for the Life Force, the condition of our body, both emotionally and physically, can relate to us what is stored in our unconscious.

From the point of view of our unconscious, aches and pains are messages. We are not their victims. In fact, they are our salvation. They are us talking to us. If we are yelling at ourselves, it is because we are desperately trying to tell ourselves where to put our focus. Pain is a red flag, an indicator that our expanding consciousness is being constricted by our outdated beliefs, our recurring emotional ruts, and their subsequent holding patterns. Pain is more than the result of a mechanical glitch; it is a plea for us to heal.

Once we accept that the root cause of our nauseated belly, our migraine headaches, our pinched nerves lies in our unconscious, we are in a position to go beyond our Band-Aid quick fixes. But in order to begin this healing, it's important for us to be able to consciously communicate with our unconscious body/mind — not so that we can control it, but so that we can let it know our intentions.

Most of us pressure and push our unconscious, trying to dictate what our ego-self wants, whether through affirmations or just plain bullying. However, the unconscious does not respond well when told what to do. When we apply pressure, the unconscious goes into a state of fight or flight, either giving pressure back or shrinking away. Even telling ourselves to relax becomes a threat, prompting defensiveness.

Instead we can use the fourth tool: Coming from Beginner's Mind, we ask a question.

Asking a Question with Beginner's Mind

When we ask a question with Beginner's Mind, we don't just ask any question. Questions such as *Am I going to be rich?* or *Is my boyfriend going to call me tonight?* or *Am I going to get that new job?* are poor questions because they assume that our intellect knows what will make us happy. In a similar way, self-pitying questions that arise from the quintessential query *Why me?* are poor questions because they create melodrama that perpetuates holding patterns, ensuring our disempowerment. We forget that the ego is a box; from inside we are unable to see beyond our preconceived borders, unable to make out the bigger picture of our lives. We are called upon to accept that it is not within the power of our ego-self to give us peace, bliss, and lightness. These emotional currents lie outside our box.

How could it be? is a better question. In fact, it is the ultimate question. By asking this question of Spirit, we presuppose that something bigger than our ego-self knows better, that our Spirit has the innate intelligence to extract for us, from the infinite permutations and combinations of the Unified Field, the perfect answer on a moment-to-moment basis. It is the question that all other questions we will find in this book point toward. To ask *How could it be?* of our Spirit is to ask for enlightenment.

Unfortunately, for most of us the ultimate answer would overwhelm our nervous systems. We would be unable to sustain or, in some cases, even recognize the feeling of enlightenment. Our nervous systems haven't been conditioned to uphold such a vibration, which is why such a lofty question can seem terra incognita.

Instead, let's start with more manageable questions, ones that have easy, direct applications, ones that recall a feeling we have already experienced: *What did it feel like when I finished that big project?* or *What did it feel like when I saw that glorious sunset last week?* or *What did it feel like to see my newborn for the first time?* Such questions illicit specific feelings drawn from specific memories. By starting with the familiar, we can step forward into the unknown from a place of safety, allowing our nervous systems to acclimatize using our own rhythm.

After we pause, breathe, and feel the weight, we ask a tailored question, and then wait with Beginner's Mind for the answer. It will come as E-motion. It will course through our tissue. Accompanying this E-motion might also be a picture, a smell, or an inner voice, which separately or in combination may produce an insight or revelation. Whichever way the unconscious manifests the answer, take it when and as it comes without judgment. To judge it, label it, or define it is to put ourselves back in our box. Stay open, receptive. The first lesson in the spiritual guidebook *A Course in Miracles* reads, "Nothing I see in this room, on this street, from this window, in this place, means anything."3 And the seventh lesson continues with, "I see only the past," teaching us to let go of all previous judgments, because when we assume we know the answer we become blind to further learning.4 Instead, by opening our perceptions we step out of our box and into a place where it is possible to truly *experience* the answer.

Some of us get confused about using recall in our questioning, asking, "How can I recall something from the past and still live in the present moment?" They find it easy to float back into a glorious memory or daydream about an imagined future. But I am not talking about transporting our consciousness into the past — that would take us off our center, our place of power. Instead, recall is used to elicit, in the here and now, the E-motion associated with a memory, while experiencing, in the here and now, the ramifications of that E-motion in the body. Again, attached might be a picture or a smell or a voice, but the power core, which is funneled into our ner-vous system via our unconscious, is the E-motion.

The tool of questioning in the form of recall can be used alongside everything else we do, not only while performing exercises from a self-help book. Consider the ramifications: During an emotionally heated discussion with our mate, we could pause, breathe, feel the weight, and ask, *How did I feel when we walked hand in hand down the beach?* During the second week of a cleansing diet when we feel ourselves sliding down the slippery slope to the kitchen cookie cupboard, we could pause, breathe, feel the weight, and ask, *How did I feel when I was full of resolve?* As we move into a pressured situation at work, we could pause, breathe, feel the weight, and ask, *What was the feeling when I handled yesterday's meeting with ease and grace?*

This is a powerful tool.

Mentastics 7: Asking a Question with Beginner's Mind

1. Stand easily with your feet shoulder-width apart. Close your eyes if it helps you to be in the moment more easily. Allow yourself to pause a moment. . . . Open the stopper to your sink full of thoughts, and watch them drain away.
2. Breathe into your belly, diaphragm, and chest as if you were opening an umbrella.

3. Feel the weight of your tailbone. Imagine grow-
    ing a tail that trails on the ground.

4. Bring your awareness to the bottoms of your
    feet. Slowly shift your weight from side to side.
    Feel the weight shift through each of the
    bones in your feet.

5. Now ask a recall question with Beginner's
    Mind, such as, *What did it feel like when my
    child came to me out of the blue and hugged
    me, saying, "I love you"*? Or ask, *What did it
    feel like when I stopped to watch that glorious
    sunset the other day?* Or ask any other recall
    question along these same lines that relates to
    a specific experience. And with Beginner's
    Mind allow yourself to pause, breathe, feel the
    weight....

6. Wait for the answer to come, and notice how
    you receive the response. Acknowledge your
    unconscious by saying something like *Thank
    you* or *Great* or *Brilliant*.

7. If you have pain or discomfort of some kind,
    you can ask your headache, sore muscles, or
    stiff joints, *What could feel softer here, more
    open?* or *What would less pressure feel like?*
    And with Beginner's Mind allow yourself to
    pause, breathe, and feel the weight....

8. Wait for the answer to come, and notice how
    you receive the response. Again, acknowledge
    your unconscious.

The tool of questioning can also be applied during a Trager session. Many practitioners use questioning like a mantra. By first maintaining presence — through pausing, breathing into their umbrella, and feeling the weight — they explore a client's holding pattern by repeatedly (and silently) asking, *How could it be?* This leads practitioners underneath the holding, opening both themselves and their clients to receive the purity of the Unified Field.

As a client, we can assist with this process. If, while a practitioner is fluffing our shoulder, or rocking our belly, or jiggling our thigh, we notice that it feels stiff and heavy, we can simply pause any spinning in our mind...take a breath into our umbrella...feel the weight of the tissue being jiggled, and inwardly ask, *How soft can you be?* We can wait with Beginner's Mind for the answer. Then we can ask again, *What can be softer than that?* And we can pause internally to notice the response. We can ask one more time: *What could be softer than even that?* And wait with open attention for the answer to come. Most often the tissue responds by opening, softening, and melting, but sometimes it expresses itself through jerks, shudders, and twitches. By asking our unconscious questions of our holding patterns throughout a Trager session, we accelerate the clearing of our body/mind conduit, thus deepening in our tissue the sensation of our conscious connection to the absolute.

An added benefit of our conscious, receptive participation is that later, after the initial effects of the session have faded, we are better able to recall the feeling of those soft, light movements we experienced on the table. So when our lower back aches, or our elbow hurts, or we're getting extra pressure from our boss, we can pause, breathe, feel the weight, and use the session as a powerful memory we can recall, opening once again to a conscious experience of the absolute.

❋

If our conscious body/mind is the captain of our ship, then the unconscious body/mind is the crew. The crew pulls the oars, sets the sails, and repairs the rudder. Without our crew on our side, we get nowhere fast. The captain can berate and flog till the mermaids sing Dixieland jazz, but until the crew members are given due respect their cooperation will be lackluster at best. They know they are irreplaceable. They know the captain can't just stop off at the next port and hire new hands. A wise captain gives his or her crew members the respect they deserve.

By asking questions of our unconscious (rather than dictating what we *think* we want), we give our crew its due. As captain, in effect we are asking our crew members to work with us. We are asking for their input, their skill, their expertise. Do they want to feel lousy, disempowered, and depressed? Of course not. By nature they are industrious folk. They want to work hard, but they also demand respect. And respect is implicit when we ask a question.

Before long a dialogue starts up. Not only do we want to communicate with our unconscious; our unconscious wants to communicate with us. By asking a question we can elicit more than just a recalled feeling. We can discover the status of our ship: what needs to be repaired and how, what maintenance requires daily attention, how a disgruntled crew member can be soothed and helped.

Questioning with Beginner's Mind gives us a way into negotiating the complexities of our ship and crew. With their expert help, a tangled physical/emotional jumble can unravel like magic, giving us clarity and ease.

Sometimes, however, as I know all too well, it is difficult to step out of our angst and sense of feeling overwhelmed and ask a question. For this very reason, it's important to cultivate the tools — pause, then breathe and feel the weight — until they become automatic. Once we are Hooked-Up, we are closer to the hub of our wheel. From here we gain some distance from our dysfunction, a distance that affords us not only the ability to ask a question, but also — and just as important — to ask it with Beginner's Mind, with open attentiveness. When we embody such an attitude when we ask our questions — such as *How could the chronic pain in my hip feel softer?* — we will receive an answer. When we ask, *What is my aching knee telling me?* we will be told. When we ask, *How would my knee feel without pain?* we will know. And when we ask for assistance in ridding ourselves of our addictions, we will be helped.

These answers can come in a variety of ways, depending on the person. Again, an answer will first and foremost come as E-motion. It will course through our tissue. Attached to this energy in motion, however, might be a picture, or a smell, or an inner voice with an important bit of data. Pay attention to these messages — they may just be the missing pieces to a lifelong puzzle.

❧

For fifteen years I smoked. I thought little about why cigarettes had become such an intimate friend. It was automatic to reach for one when I confronted a difficult situation. Our partnership was a ritual: the shaft between my fingers, the filter against my lips, the flash of flame, the glowing ember, the deep warm inhalation, the billowing out-breath, the surge of nicotine, over and over. . . .

A cigarette provided deep, consistent comfort. It did not ask me to change into a better person or live up to a higher standard. It did not judge. It accepted me as I was, but for a price. A high price. My money out-of-pocket was exorbitant. My lungs had become congested. My deep breathing, labored. Before long I had symptoms of adult asthma. I had to stop. I knew it.

A thousand times I had quit, or so it seemed. I was ashamed of my failures, disgusted by my inability to change. But the lure of our intimacy always managed to reel me back in. None of my strategies made any difference. The cold-turkey approach of denying myself comfort for weeks merely caused the elastic band of my dysfunction to sling me back into my addiction — only deeper. Trying to slowly cut back the amount I smoked was a slippery slope: Some minor crisis always made me lose my grip. Just as ineffective was using nicotine gum as a replacement; I'd end up chewing and smoking at the same time!

I had known about the Trager tools, of course, but I balked at the starting gate. I had shied away from using them because I was afraid to lose my intimate friend. I was afraid of who I'd be without a cigarette. Knowing what I was *supposed* to do wasn't enough. My dysfunction was stronger than my knowledge.

Only years of consistent failure and deteriorating health humbled me enough to gather the courage to attempt the Trager way. Rather than trying to control the situation by applying strategies and products, I decided to explore what it would feel like if I didn't smoke, using the tool of questioning while in the present moment.

Once I'd made this decision, it took no time at all for an urge to well up. My lungs yearned for nicotine. "No!" I said automatically. But this usual tactic only escalated my craving as the claws of the nicotine monster clamped down on my chest.

"No!" I commanded again.

Regardless, incessant thoughts pushed their way through my resolve: *I deserve a cigarette. I've work hard. I should get a reward. One won't hurt me. I'll smoke only half. . . . Wait a minute. Pause. . . .*

I took a moment, just a moment, and slowed down the speeding car of my mind. I let go the reins of addiction. Stopped. I had hoped there might be a short moment of peace in this pause, some small distance created from my cravings, but instead I burst into tears. Not the lone tear of a Hollywood love story, but unabashed and uncontrolled bawling for ten minutes. When I was finished, I wiped my eyes, blew my nose, and discovered my craving had left.

Twenty minutes later, however, while I was washing the dishes, the urge reasserted itself. Before the momentum of the craving overwhelmed me, though, I remembered to use the tools. I paused, breathed into my umbrella, felt the weight of the sudsy teacup in my hand. In response, some of my resolve returned and with as much innocence as I could muster, I asked inwardly, *What would it feel like if I didn't smoke?* My chest lifted and opened. The haze in my head began to clear. Immediately following on the heels of this clarity was another question: *Do I really want to be a non-smoker?*

My chest caved in; my stomach sank. A feeling of dread drained through me. Attached were pictures of the few holier-than-thou nonsmokers I knew. Their judgments had brought me to my knees more times than I wanted to recall. If that was what it meant for me to be a nonsmoker, I wanted no part of it. *But could I become like that?* I wondered. *No*, came the immediate reply. That picture of a nonsmoker was an old, erroneous belief. My zealous nature, I realized, was fulfilled during my early years of TM. *Well, then*, I continued to question, *if I'm not going to become a zealot, who would I be if I didn't smoke?*

A light spaciousness floated into my body, expanded into my chest, and swirled down to my toes. I breathed into this feeling, felt the weight of it, and, in so doing, began to anchor it into my awareness.

Later, while pondering this new experience, I realized I had previously chosen to identify with the label "smoker." I had forgotten that I was the observer of my addiction. Smoking did not define me. I was not a "smoker." I was a person . . . who smoked.

This was a revelation. The *ah-ha* lit up not only my mind but also my body — all the way down through my belly to my feet. It was not just a mental construct but a feeling as well, and this feeling opened up a little distance between my old friend cigarettes and me.

In the following days when I had a craving, I would observe

myself being pulled into the identification of a "smoker." Sometimes the force of this identification was so strong that all I could do was put my head in my hands and cry a river. But after my tears subsided, I would pause, take a cleansing breath, and feel the weight of my feet on the floor. Continuing to Hook-Up to the Unified Field in this way, I would innocently ask more and more precise questions of Spirit to peel away deeper and deeper layers of this dysfunction — a process that took several weeks.

What am I really feeling? was one of the later questions I was prompted to ask myself in order to move through the feeling of hollowness invading my chest and belly. And as I waited with Beginner's Mind, a further understanding permeated my brain: *I was grieving for the loss of an old friend.* Without judging it or pushing it away, I allowed this feeling of grief to flow through me, washing away some of my attachment.

Later, when cravings again gnawed at my guts, I continued to ask, *What am I really feeling?* This question helped me explore what was underneath my nicotine monster. One might think that the answer to the same question would remain the same, but it didn't. It evolved. I eventually discovered that one of the switches that triggered my need to reach for my old pal cigarettes was the belief that I was inadequate to the task at hand. Bad news, unresolved conflict, and unfamiliar situations and people would all make me long for nicotine.

Over the weeks as I dug deeper using my tools, the questions I had been asking Spirit distilled to: *If I had never become a cigarette addict, then what is this feeling about?* To my surprise it had to do with my never-ending search to consciously feel the Life Force flowing throughout my tissue. Cigarettes were a soother to pacify a deep emptiness in my belly and chest. When I was unable or unwilling to accept the constant unconditional love of Spirit, I substituted nicotine.

From that moment on, I used the feeling of yearning for a cigarette as a trigger to prompt me to pause... breathe... feel the weight of my tailbone, and ask, *What does the unconditional love of Spirit feel like?* In answer, my body would become soft and fluffy, buoyant and playful, almost ethereal, and yet safely anchored. In this way a nicotine craving became my ally; each time it dug in its claws, it would remind me to use my tools and recall the feeling of unconditional love. Within a week I effortlessly stopped smoking.

I haven't picked up a cigarette since.

❧

By pausing, breathing, feeling weight, and questioning, we not only become aware of an E-motion but we also receive a revelation. Our unconscious (if we ask) can peel away the layers of our onion and uncover the dynamics around our habits, our addictions, or any other serious (or not-so-serious) inner conflict.

Most of us have forgotten that we have a choice about the emotions that color our lives. We have forgotten what the connection to the Unified Field feels like. Our everyday lives have taken us more and more out of that place of infinite wisdom and into the realm of reaction. We think we are machines running on the same principles as they do. As we move faster and faster and faster, we lose the conscious connection to the Life Force. Soon our Spirit is no longer nourished. A feeling of indefinable loss manifests deep inside our belly and around our solar plexus — that vague space in our guts that we don't often take the time to acknowledge until it gives us problems. In the meantime, we habitually try to satisfy this emptiness with junk food, more clothes, a new car, or more serious addictions.

As the layers of our onion peel away through questioning and we begin to receive different feeling experiences, the expressions of our addiction, habit, or chronic pain sometimes change. The pain we used to have in a shoulder is now in a hip or foot. We stop biting our nails only to replace it with clearing our throats. We stop smoking but can't get enough chocolate into our mouths. These new messages tell us there is more to uncover — that we have even deeper areas where we have held on to an outmoded belief. We realize subtler and subtler layers of our holding patterns. The deeper we go in this process, the clearer our conscious communication with Spirit becomes, causing the nervous system to strengthen and enabling us to accept more of Spirit, which strengthens the nervous system even further — a powerful feedback loop.

Questioning with Beginner's Mind while in the present moment is another one of the simple array of tools that lift away the layers of our dysfunction, helping us to remain empowered while traversing the winding road to a better way of life. Even when we find ourselves feeling down, we can gently cultivate presence, which automatically gives us the strength to ask a simple question that can change the momentum of our low state, bringing us into joy.

Using the tools of pausing, breathing into our umbrella,

feeling the weight, and asking a question with Beginner's Mind keeps us away from self-pity, self-doubt, and concerns over the opinions of others. These tools keep us making good choices. They enrich our appreciation of life and attract the kind of energy, people, and relationships that support our authentic selves. They are the foundation to living 100 percent in the relative and 100 percent in the absolute.

CHAPTER ELEVEN

Trusting Ourselves Not to Know

I do not know what this, or anything means
And so I do not know how to respond to it
I will not use my past as a light to guide me now
I will step aside and let You lead the way.

This holy instant would I give to You
Be You in charge
For I would follow You
Certain that Your direction gives me peace.

— *A COURSE IN MIRACLES*

I n the previous two chapters we learned how to utilize tools that consciously and effectively connect our body/mind to the intelligence of the Unified Field. Our next step is to deepen our understanding of Beginner's Mind, of the multiple facets around the idea of waiting with innocence for the

Life Force to answer. What does it mean to have the innocence of a beginner when doing the same job for fifteen years? What does it mean to have innocence when we have been vacuuming the same floor for twenty? How about when looking at the same face across the breakfast table for more times than we can remember? And what does it mean to have innocence when looking in the mirror?

It means loosening the reins of what we *thought* we knew. It means opening up to a world that continues to unfold on all levels. It means trusting ourselves not to know what is going to happen next.

To accomplish this, we are called upon to trust that if we are in presence the information we receive from the Life Force is, in that moment, tailor-made for us. This kind of trust is difficult for our ego-self because the Life Force exists outside its box, outside the sense of identity that says, *I am an individual. I am separate from.* Our ego-self does not trust because it rarely recognizes that it is part of a whole from which all support comes. In addition, our ego-self gets caught up in the daily spin of events and forgets that it has much less responsibility than it believes. It thinks it must keep us safe, create goals and fulfill them, thereby controlling the path of our life. But on a fundamental level it has only one of two choices to make: to be present, or not to be present. That is its dilemma.

The choice we make creates a domino effect, leading us toward a particular way of being. When we choose to be present, we take the path of least resistance to manifesting the answer to the ultimate question, *How could it be?* Veils peel away, revealing our authentic self. More and more our identity aligns itself with the whole: 100 percent of the relative (our sense of self) and 100 percent of the absolute (our sense of Spirit).

However, most of us, consciously or unconsciously, have chosen not to be present. Therefore, our default choice is to relive the past, recirculating it in our mind over and over again in countless variations, and then projecting it out into an extrapolated future. This choice soon becomes a habit, a way of being that, unfortunately, blocks much of our support from the Life Force, making our ego-self assume there is nothing other than the past to guide us. With this assumption, our identity aligns itself with the past.

Our remembered past, however, has a basic limitation. It gives us only a single point of view, a single camera with which to record the world. How much sense does it make to base all of our beliefs on a single point of view — a view that by its very nature is incomplete? If our past tells us a teapot is only for brewing tea, we won't consider that it has other potential uses — as a flowerpot, for example, or as a place for storing petty cash. If we failed in business before, we assume we lack business sense; we assume we are failures. If we had an evangelical upbringing, we assume our religion will save everyone. If our past tells us something is true, we assume it is: Men are poor listeners. Women are flaky. Black people are violent. White people are prejudiced. A turban equals a terrorist.

The accumulation of our judgments (and the judgments of others) regarding our varying successes, failures, pains, and joys becomes a filter that allows in only a fraction of the information available in the moment. By assuming that the microamount of information we receive through these filters is reliable, accurate, and all there is, we invest our identity with it, creating our box, making it an inflexible set of parameters by which we interpret ourselves, those around us, and the world at large.

To a degree, making assumptions helps us navigate our life smoothly — it can be useful, there's no doubt. But making assumptions is also a double-edged sword because attached to assumptions are expectations. Expectations are the past thrown in linear lines out into the future. They automatically push us, subtly but powerfully, to re-create yet another variation of the same old painting, using the same old colors. Of course, we don't re-create the past on purpose. I don't recall ever hearing anyone stand up and say, "Hey, I love alcoholics. I want to live with three, one after another. Abusive relationships? Great. Give me half a dozen. And while you're at it, throw in a couple of tyrannical bosses." Nevertheless, we do re-create the past, over and over. We re-create the past because when we are not present our awareness becomes backward oriented, our thoughts a recirculation of our previous thoughts. The only other choice we can make if we want to create something new, to become more, to embody our dreams, is to loosen our expectations and choose to live in the present moment.

To some this idea of trusting something that is constantly on the move, constantly changing, may not sound any better than trusting a projection of the past. But, remember, this constant motion and change is intelligent. This intelligence is the foundation of the perennial nature of the cosmos. And, believe it or not, it's safe. In fact, it's the safest place for our ego to be. Despite what past conditioning might say, by riding the enfolding waves of the Life Force we will not only survive but flourish. If we trust ourselves to Spirit, the intelligent nature of the Life Force will give us the perfect response to any situation we may find ourselves in. Such responses, over time, will build and manifest for us the right job that explores our creative potential, the best relationship that supports our growth, the lifestyle that is perfect for our authentic self.

A Practitioner's Inner Dialogue with a Neck

The following is an example of an experienced Trager practitioner who cares deeply for his clients and, despite being taught to "stay out of his own way," cannot help but invest expectations around his ability to heal. In other words, underneath his training he still thinks he has to *fix* his clients. He assumes too much responsibility, creating expectations that subtly push for an outcome, causing the client unconsciously to push back. Without realizing it, the practitioner's ego-self has stopped trusting the intelligent flow of Life Force. This creates the same old picture: He leads a client only so far down the road of healing before hitting a wall, a wall he is only now finding a door through.

Session #7

Hi there, neck. How are you today? Softer... good. The Mentastics are helping. How would it feel to take this softness deeper in? Hmm, something's still here... around the occiput... the subtle holding I detected last session. Still feels anchored, too. Let's experiment with nodding the head . . . no, that's not working. All right, let's elongate the spine. . . . Hmm . . . that helps a bit, but the holding's still there. . . .

Session #8

Hi, neck. Hmm . . . you feel a little looser today. Head's moving well, too . . . oh, but not so much here. You're still holding around your occiput — this is my third week butting up against this. It's your control center, I know now. What magic is going to undo you? Maybe this new move. . . . Oh no, it's tightening up even more. Better go lighter. Lighter still . . . ah, that's better. Not great, but better. . . .

Session #9

Here we are again, neck. Hmm . . . feeling a bit dense today. What would softer be like? Yes, that's it . . . yeah, good. How could this softness go deeper in? Beautiful . . . yes . . . keep going. . . . Oh, but there's that holding again. The same spot, the control center. Come on; let me in. Unlock. I know you can. Come on, come on. All your chest problems would evaporate if I could just pick your lock. Why won't you let me? Am I doing something wrong?

Session #10

Neck, we dance again. Hmm . . . how are you this time? Your outer tissue yields; your inner core resists. I know

I'm reaching you; why won't you unlock? What are you afraid of? How can I make you feel safe? Nothing I'm doing seems to be working. What can I do?

Step back; that's what I can do. Yes, right off the table. Pause...breathe into my umbrella...feel my weight shifting. Ahhhh...Hook-Up...yes...

Let go of what I think I know, what I think I should do next....Trust the Life Force. Pause... breathe...feel my weight....How should it be?

Your hip. It's calling me. The right side. Hmm, I would have expected the shoulder. Oh well, let's explore.

Okay, what's here? Some resistance in the sacroiliac. Oops, I'm pushing. Don't try. Remember: no effort, no agenda. Trust. Good, some release. Now what could be half this effort? And half of that? Yum. And half again? Yes, that feeling...yes...

Okay, step away again. Pause...breathe...feel my weight....Where am I drawn to next? The neck. Really? All right, let's explore again. No agenda.

Hi again, neck. You know it's me, and you tense. Why are you afraid? Is it me? Have I been pushing? I have, haven't I? I've pushed, and you've pushed back. Okay, then, what would it feel like to allow you to be how you truly are? Yes, that light feeling...good...and what is lighter than that? Beautiful...and what would it feel like to be free? Ah, yes...that's the one...so deep ...yes, yes...I stopped trying to control the outcome and you unlocked.

Trust: It's the key.

With an attitude of trust, this practitioner stepped away from his assumption that he knew what his client's tissue wanted. Applying a stance of *not knowing* erased his preconceived ideas of how the tissue *should* be (only Spirit knows that!) and primed his awareness to receive, opening him to new information, allowing his client to enter the next level of healing.

Going with the Flow

Having trust in the knowledge and intelligence of the Life Force means going with the flow even if it's not what we expect. This applies not only to Trager practitioners, but to everyone, be they writers or waiters, fathers or mothers, bankers or doctors, clerks or gardeners. Staying in the moment and trusting ourselves not to know what will happen next can be especially difficult when there is perceived pressure on a situation. I remember the night before teaching my first workshop. . . .

❧

I sat at my desk fretting. My mind went round and round over what I wanted to have happen during my first class the next day. My plan was to have the students start by sitting in a circle; then I would introduce myself and get their names. I'd talk about Trager and Mentastics, and tell them about Dr. Trager's life. Oh, and I couldn't forget to tell the story about him and Mickey Martin. But I also had to avoid going into too much detail — that would put me behind schedule. I had so much to do. How was I going to fit it all in? I had to put my notes in order: How else was I going to remember to say and do all that I had planned? Best not have my nose in my notes, though. Maybe I should make up cue cards — that might help. But it was so late already; was I ever going to get some sleep?

With the tides of feeling overwhelmed rising to my chest, I mindfully took an in-breath. *Where are my feet?* I thought. *There they are. I'm all right. Feel the weight. It will all get done.*

Long after midnight, my exhausted body crawled under the covers. My mind longed for oblivion. But I couldn't get comfortable. When I lay on my right side, my shoulder ached. When I rolled onto my left, my neck felt kinked. No matter how I positioned my body, I couldn't sleep. I flipped onto my back and jerked the quilt up to my neck. *Okay,* I fumed, *pause, breathe, feel the weight of my tailbone. My jaw is tight; I'd better feel the weight of that too. Now, ask a question: What would it feel like to be asleep? Wait for the answer. Again. Pause, breathe, feel the weight. What does asleep feel like? Wait for the answer. And again. Damn!*

It wasn't working. I was still wide-awake. What could I do? A warm bath was out of the question. Even the idea of brewing chamomile tea exhausted me. I was just too tired to get up. All I could do was lie there and do it again.

Okay, slowly *this time . . .*

Pause . . . (I imagined my thoughts were like helium balloons I released).

Breathe . . . (I pictured my chest as an umbrella smoothly opening and closing).

Feel the weight . . . (I rolled my head gently from side to side, feeling my jaw shift).

What would it feel like to let go? . . . (I trusted and left the door to my body/mind ajar).

Pause . . . (my bed turned into a cloud; I sank into its softness).

Breathe . . . (my umbrella became lighter, wider, fuller).

Feel the wei—. . .

At 7:00 A.M. my clock radio clicked on. "Tickets go on sale in an hour," a pushy baritone voice boomed, "so stop what you're doing and hurry on down!" For some reason the volume was cranked. "Don't be disappointed. By noon they'll be long gone!"

My right hand smacked down the snooze button and then flopped back to my side. My strength had been stolen from me in the night. I was glued to the mattress, dizzy and disoriented. My head throbbed. My joints ached. Remnants of stress dreams buzzed about my head: lost keys, empty chairs, a skipping CD player, irate students, people wanting a refund. How was I going to make it through the day? I had a class to teach — in this, there was no choice.

Somehow, I managed to swing my legs over the edge of the bed and rise to my feet. My legs went rubbery. The butterflies in my stomach awoke. A wave of nausea fluttered up from my belly. I was teetering on the edge of a steep cliff. I felt for my safety line — it had become automatic. Brushing my teeth, I paused and breathed into my umbrella. Getting dressed, I felt the weight of my limbs slide through my clothes. Picking up the first of the boxes to be taken to the car, I asked, *What does light feel like?* I paused, and almost immediately my tissue seemed buoyant, the boxes emptier. By the time I had driven out of my driveway I had found home base. I realized I *did* have a choice: I could give in to feeling overwhelmed, *or* I could stay present and trust Spirit.

One by one the students walked into the dance studio I had rented for the class. Some I had seen before; others looked as if they were new to Trager. As the room filled I mentally reviewed my notes from the night before. I had wanted to start with a brief circle so I could introduce myself, get to know the participants, and then explain Trager and Mentastics. But things were different now; I had to acknowledge I was no longer that person sitting at my desk and planning the perfect class. I was nervous, tired, and fragile. It took all my resources just to choose presence. I no longer had the energy to stay in control.

When all the students had arrived, the room resonated with the general buzz of pre-class activity. A few renewed old acquaintances as they got comfortable on the many throw cushions. Some searched for places to stow their belongings. Others exchanged introductions over the snack table. The group needed focus.

"Everyone… everyone… please, can I have your attention?"

But no one heard. It was like talking to a wall. Their bodies were there, but their minds were not present.

"Everyone… your attention please."

No one was responding. Was I invisible? What little confidence I had started a downward spiral. I was losing the class, and we hadn't even started! Luckily, because I had been consciously fostering presence all morning, home base wasn't far off. Once again, I paused. Breathed into my umbrella. Felt the weight of my tailbone. And made a different choice.

Although I had not planned it, I skipped the introduction, and started up the CD I had brought, which immediately drew everyone's attention. Then, I began to walk about the room. "Join me," I said, and soon they were all on their feet.

As we walked, I noticed the tiredness in my own body, a dull gray that murmured a solitary note. It was easy to feel the weight of my limbs in such a state. Although I was exhausted, this awareness deepened my presence. From there I asked an inward question: *What could feel lighter?* Instantly, much of my tiredness washed away. My perception cleared. I felt a discord in the room. Noticed a lack of attention — a kind of aimlessness to their walking.

· "Become aware of the bottoms of your feet," I instructed. "This will ground your energy and help you to *arrive* in the room — connect you to the here and now." Their walking slowed, became more deliberate. "Take your time," I said. "Notice how your feet connect with the floor." I could sense their inner attention waking up as we walked around the dance studio. "Now imagine you have a long tail. It can be any kind of tail you want, as long as it trails on the floor. Feel its weight behind you. Good..."

Along with the giggles and snickers, I noticed a subtle change in their posture. Their bellies no longer scrunched into their pelvises; their lower backs lengthened. "Next, imagine a thin thread coming down from the heavens, attached to the top of your head directly above your ears. This is your skyhook. It supports you from above while your tail supports you from below." As a group, their movements became fluid, their gaits purposeful, their postures upright. The fog in their expressions cleared. A sense of lightness radiated through the room. I gave them time to bask in this feeling.

A smile crept upon my face. It was working! We moved on. "Let's take a moment to pause, now. That's right. Pause. Stop your doing, even your thinking." The room went silent. "Breathe into your belly and chest as if you were opening an umbrella...and breathe out closing your umbrella." A long collective sigh reverberated around the room. I looked at the changed faces. Everyone seemed brighter, clearer, more present. "You are now connected to the energy of the Life Force. This energy is the food that nourishes our body/mind."

By becoming present and trusting in the Life Force to give me direction, I was able to teach these students through a body experience what I had planned to tell them in words while in circle. When we finally settled into our chairs, this experience became the basis for clearer intellectual understanding.

During our morning break I wandered off by myself to the oversized windows that lined one wall and gazed down at the traffic coursing along Rideau Street. I patted myself on the back for getting through the hardest part — the beginning. Puffed up by this success, I found myself planning what we were going to do next, my mind running on as if I was the choreographer of a dance. Suddenly, panic crept along my spine and into my chest. My breathing became rapid and shallow. But as I zoomed off into an imagined future, I heard, over my right shoulder, the word *grounded* coming from a student at the snack table. It gave me pause. It brought me back to my original commitment: to trust not to know what was going to happen next.

I tuned into the class's conversations. Many of the students were talking about how hard it was to keep their heads above water, how hard it was to raise children in these turbulent times, how hard it was to keep their family units together. What a struggle!

I felt the heaviness of their conversations. It seemed as if they had forgotten what soft felt like. What effortlessness felt like. What trust felt like. I paused, and felt the weight of this discovery. A brilliant idea came to mind. When the break ended, I invited everyone back to the circle. As they gathered, I scanned their faces and asked, "So, what is soft? What does soft feel like?"

Several gave definitions. Others used similes, "It's like..."

"Let's experiment with something," I suggested. "Let's pile up these throw cushions and explore this concept of soft." In a minute we had a small mountain of cushions in the center of the room. Like kids we started to play. We frolicked on them and experienced their softness. We tossed them around and felt their lightness. We walked on them to further absorb the feeling of softness into our bodies. Before long, this exercise turned into a lesson on trust. The class divided into pairs. Each partner blindfolded the other and led that person over the mountain of pillows. Our fun escalated. People squealed with delight... and fear.

Then, I started to worry. Were things getting out of control? Were people learning what they needed to know? It was up to me. I was the one in charge. I closed my eyes. Paused. Took a deep breath. Felt the weight of my tail. Asked, *Where do we go from here?* In response to my asking this question of Spirit, the peak of high energy declined. The class intuitively followed my lead. In the space of a few breaths, the student's emotions transitioned to a soft glow. Soon everyone drifted down, like snowflakes, onto a pillow.

Revelations emerged: "I never knew what it felt like to melt with every step. Mmm. I want more of that in my life," said one.

Another piped up, "Trust has been a big issue of mine. Letting go feels so freeing."

Still another exclaimed, "I did it! I actually trusted someone enough to let her be in charge while I walked the pillows blindfolded. It was like walking over coals."

Trusting in the intelligence of the Life Force gave me flexibility that allowed me to playfully explore different ways that easily and effortlessly relayed the messages I wanted the class to learn. Coming from this place of trust, my role became one of facilitator. I gave up needing to know what would happen next; I let the Life Force guide me. Staying present to the immediate vibe in the class, I was able to address the students' specific dynamics. In the end, my first class was a success. Everyone went home fulfilled.

❧

Commitment to an attitude of not knowing encompasses subtle layers of trust that may take time to unwind. It requires, first, that we trust that we are going to receive from Spirit something that has validity to our life, and, second, that we trust that what we receive will come to us from a place of love and compassion, regardless of whether it's what we expect.

Unfortunately, what many of us call trust is really based on whether or not the expectations of our ego-self are met. When the result of such pseudotrust does not fall within this narrow bandwidth, we feel betrayed. "If the Life Force is so intelligent, why did I have to go through that heartbreak? Why didn't I get the job I wanted? Why didn't I get the sale?" Disappointment occurs when our ego-self tries to control the world *out there.*

The ego-self, unable to relate easily to the nonlinear nature of the Life Force, rarely considers there might be a better way. It's hard for the ego to trust anything outside its box. *How can I trust something I can't understand?* it says. *How can I put stock in a mystery?* The ego wants to understand now. It wants a lightbulb to flick on, accompanied by a solid plan and goals it can implement. It wants neat-and-tidy static answers because it believes that's where safety lies. What the ego needs to remember, however, is that it cannot accurately perceive outside its box. Therefore, attempting to control any situation in order to manifest preconceived expectations becomes an extremely dicey and overwhelming task.

As a result, the ego feels caught between a rock and a hard place. To align itself with the past means living through illusion, but to trust the Life Force is to jump off a cliff and "boldly go where no one has gone before," to use the phrase from the *Star Trek* series. Why would we want to trust in something constantly on the move? Because that is life. We change; the world changes. Change is constant. Our knowledge evolves as we evolve. "Knowledge is structured in consciousness," Maharishi Mahesh Yogi has stated.[5] How it *is* today may not be how it *will be* tomorrow. Our perceptions continually change as we mold and shape our sculpture, as we paint our painting. Each mark of the chisel, each stroke of the brush alters how we see ourselves and the world around us. Life is multidimensional and never ending. There is never a time when we have "arrived." Reality-based answers, true answers, are process oriented, not static and definitive.

To counter the fear of jumping off the cliff into the unknown, we need to anchor back into the energy of the Unified Field. From the past there is only memory to comfort and guide us, but in the present moment there is the blissful feeling of Spirit — it's real, it's physical, you *can* feel it. If we focus within, trusting in our tools, the manifestation of our life happens easily and naturally, in line with our authentic self. Stepping out of our box becomes effortless and, above all, safe. When our ego-self follows this flow, it aligns itself with Spirit. That is its job — its real job: to choose to use the tools to Hook-Up. This is where the ego's true power lies.

Choosing to live without expectations instead of sticking to the tried-and-true from our past is making a choice to *not know*. This requires trust.

The fifth tool is trusting ourselves not to know.

I trust you.
I trust the sun will rise tomorrow.
I trust the universe.
I trust in All That Is.
I trust myself not to know what is going to happen next.

CHAPTER TWELVE

Finding Our Rhythm

The last of the six tools we will use to actualize the source of our being into the fabric of our daily lives is finding our rhythm. The first four tools give us something *to do*: When we pause, we apply the brakes; when we breathe, we move our umbrella in and out; when we feel the weight, we play with gravity; and when we ask a question, we put forth an intention in a specific way. These four are the active tools, designed to open up our body/mind to Spirit. The last two — trusting ourselves not to know, and finding our rhythm — foster receptivity.

Both aspects — active and receptive — are necessary. Otherwise the circuit is not complete, the cycle not perpetual. Such is the nature of a self-sustaining system. We need both a ying and a yang. Creation is cyclical. We all live and die. The sun rises and sets. The moon waxes and wanes. The tides of the ocean ebb and flow. Our lungs inhale and exhale.

The heart expands and contracts. Similarly, we need to receive as well as to act.

The question is: How can our receptivity become clear, effortless, and efficient? First, by strengthening our trust that Spirit has the right answers for the situation at hand. And, second, by finding and accepting our personal rhythm, we become conscious of the pace at which Spirit manifests in our body/mind and life. This means getting in touch with our individual ebbs and flows, and accepting how quickly or slowly we naturally do things: the rate at which we move through space, take in information, and process it, as well as the rate at which we interact with the rest of the world.

Finding Our Sweet Spot

It is like dancing — first you pause and listen
to the music, then the rhythm within you pulsates
to the rhythm of the music, your body begins swaying
and before you realize it, you're on your feet dancing.
But it doesn't have to be music for there is a rhythm to
everything in life and if you will just get the feel *of that*
rhythm, there are no limits to what your body will do.[6]

— MILTON TRAGER

When we innocently explore, and then discover and accept, our personal rhythm within, we have found our *sweet spot*, that one place on the drum of our soul where the music of life is sweeter, fuller, and lighter — and where the harmonious correlation of all our parts move as one. When we find this sweet spot, we have found our personal rhythm — the final piece in our toolbox.

At workshops I often get the participants dancing to music that has within it multiple rhythms in order to explore the body's urge to move. I get the group to use the first five tools to assist them in exploring the sixth. I get them to pause, breathe, and feel the weight, then ask the question *What movement does my body want to do right now?* Then I tell them to wait with Beginner's Mind for the answer to come.

I encourage them to trust not to know what will happen next as they turn their attention inward and listen to what a shoulder or leg or neck or any other part of the body has to say and how it wants to move. They are not to move until they *hear* an answer, and *hearing* could come in any form. It could be an urge or a thought or a physical sensation.

I also remind them that they do not know ahead of time how a particular part of their bodies want to move. I encourage them not to go to the past for their usual way of moving but to stay in a state of *not knowing*. They have to be still within, connected, Hooked-Up, in order to hear what the different parts of their bodies are saying. If they are not hearing anything, then I suggest they rest with open attention until they receive something from the flow of the Life Force.

In other words, I want them to stop assuming that they know how their bodies want to move and become innocent explorers who are listening to find out what their bodies are actually telling them. Remaining innocent introduces them to their selves in a totally different way.

The following exercise will give us a taste of our personal rhythm. If we listen to our bodies with innocent attentiveness, they will clearly communicate to us what our most efficient pace is for the moment.

Mentastics 8: Finding Rhythms Within

1. Put on a record, tape, or CD, or tune in to some great music on your computer or radio, or just listen to the music of life. Be in bare or stocking feet if possible. Stand easily with your feet shoulder-width apart.
2. Close your eyes.
3. Allow yourself to pause. . . .
4. Breathe into your belly, diaphragm, and chest as if you were opening an umbrella.
5. Feel the weight of your tailbone by imagining a tail that trails on the ground.
6. Bring your awareness to the bottoms of your feet; imagine you are growing roots into the earth.
7. Pause . . . breathe . . . feel the weight of a part of your body.
8. Ask yourself, *What movement does my body want to do right now?* With Beginner's Mind, wait for the answer to come.
9. Your body may want to sway to the music, it may want to jump up and down, or it may just want to twitch — it doesn't matter. If you're not hearing your body speak, then just rest with open attention.
10. After the movement fulfills itself, come to a pause. . . . Breathe. . . . Feel the weight.
11. Wait with open attention for the next message that urges you to move.
12. Continue in this state of not knowing, inviting yourself to remain open to receive.

Many factors combine to create our personal rhythm. It's like making a pot of soup; the flavor and thickness vary, depending on the ingredients we add to it. Our height and weight play a part. A wave of motion looks much different on a short, chubby arm than on a long, lean one. Our bone density matters too. A bird with hollow bones moves differently than an ox with dense bones. Our holding patterns are also important. No matter what we weigh on the scales, if we are holding in our chest and spine they will seem denser and heavier as they move through space than if these areas were flexible and fluid. Aging is another significant factor. As people grow older their rhythms slow; their speech and movement mellow. When we were children, the pace at which we skipped down the street, played with our toys, ate our lunches, and put on our clothes, differed from how, at middle age, we go for a walk, clean our houses, and dance with our partners.

Yet another factor is our environment. People from the tropics generally have a rhythm that differs from that of people in a temperate climate. "Aloha" conjures up a different feeling than "Hi there!" or "G'day, g'day." To add to this, each personality has a unique rhythm. We have all encountered the "fast talker," or "the contemplator," or "the step-by-step person," to mention only a few. Still another spice to add to the soup is the degree of our conscious awareness. Relatively speaking, our rhythm slows as our consciousness awakens because we are no longer going on automatic; we experience the world as a bigger, more complex organism, and respond with greater mindfulness.

Moreover, within each of us a variety of rhythms are all happening simultaneously. There are the rhythms of the internal body: chemistry, blood flow, heartbeat, sleep stages, and, for women, menstrual cycles — the list goes on.

In addition, there are varying rhythms to different parts of the body: A hand has a quicker rhythm than an arm; comparing the rhythm of the toes to that of the legs is like comparing a chickadee to a crane. Then there are the rhythms of our thoughts and how we process information. Some days we — *bing-bing-bing* — process ideas and emotions right away, while on other days our assimilation curve is much longer. Only by adding up all these rhythms do we come to our overall personal rhythm.

Trager practitioners teach their clients how to find their personal rhythm by giving them a feeling of what it is like to move at their own pace. Kinesthetic experience is the key here. We can't figure out our rhythm intellectually; the recipe is too complex — not to mention nonlinear. It evolves as we do. Instead, the most effective route is to get to know what rhythm *feels* best. A Trager practitioner does this by using the inherent rhythm in the client's tissue as a wave that carries the question of *How could it be?* to the client's unconscious mind. This question is automatically answered by the Life Force and subsequently transferred as sensation to the various muscles, ligaments, and tendons. Afterward, the client can recall and reinforce the memory of this rhythm.

Mentastics, of course, are another great way to get in touch with our rhythms. In this chapter, Mentastics 8 (using music) provided an experience of this. There are many Mentastics that can help. Mentastics 9 offers a simple example we can use to find our rhythm using the range of motion of a leg when we are sitting on a flat surface with our legs out in front of us. Using the soft grip of our palm on the outside of our thigh, we can roll the leg inward and allow it to return unimpeded. If we perform this simple movement while in presence, the leg starts to move with less and less effort. Soon, it feels as if it is flowing with gravity, rather than against it. Before long the rhythm of this movement brings our whole body/mind into Hook-Up.

Such movement explorations can become as effortless as a fish swimming through water or an eagle soaring on an updraft — we are only as limited as our imagination when accessing what could be soft, free, and light. Experiment on your own leg.

Mentastics 9:
Finding Your Rhythm Using Your Legs

1. Sit on the floor or another firm surface with your legs hip-width apart and stretched out before you.
2. Allow yourself to pause. . . .
3. Breathe into your umbrella. Feel it.
4. Notice the weight of your tailbone on the floor.
5. Now, slurp up the tissue on the outside of your midthigh with a widely opened palm and fingers and roll your whole leg inward. Let go of the push while still maintaining contact with your leg, and feel your leg rolling back.
6. Play with different rhythms until you come to one that goes deepest, the one that feels light and playful with minimal effort. This will be

your sweet spot for the rhythm of your leg for this present moment.

7. As you perform these Mentastics, you may want to ask yourself, *What could be half that effort?* In this way you engage the rhythm and knowledge of the Life Force, prompting the feeling experience to go even deeper.

Now let's explore a similar process using our arms and shoulders.

Mentastics 10: Finding Your Rhythm Using Your Arms and Shoulders

1. Stand with your feet comfortably spaced the width of your shoulders, or sit feeling your tailbone on a chair.
2. Pause.... Breathe into your umbrella.... Feel the weight of your tailbone.
3. Leading with your shoulder, bend your torso slightly to the side. (Be careful, though, not to collapse your rib cage into your waist by leaning over too far. Most people find that as soon as the upper arm is no longer in contact with the rib cage, that's far enough.)
4. Imagine a string attached to your elbow, pulling it up an inch or two. Allow your forearm to just hang there. Feel the weight of your hand.

5. Now, gently but freely let your arm drop. Notice the rebound as it bounces back up.
6. Do this again. Your elbow is lifted by the string an inch or two. Feel the weight of your hand. Gently but playfully let it fall. Notice the bounce.
7. Continue to playfully lift and drop, exploring the rhythm of this movement until you come to a place where your arm bounces back up as if by itself.
8. As you are performing this movement, ask yourself, *What could be lighter here?* or *How could I use half the effort?* Allow the answer to come to you.

We can use rhythm as a tool to help us stay in the present moment. It is a receptive tool. We do not choose our personal rhythm, but rather allow it to emerge from Spirit through presence. The ability to recognize and then allow this rhythm into our conscious body/mind is a process similar to all the other tools. It often takes time and the by-now-familiar "measles principle" (we can "catch it" by being in the presence of someone who already has it). If we stay in the here and now, pausing, breathing into our umbrella, feeling the weight of a part of the body, asking a question such as *What could be lighter?* and then waiting with innocent trust for an answer, we need only observe the rhythm that tends to emerge — this will be our personal rhythm. Trust this pace.

For virtually every situation a rhythm will emerge that

works for us. Unfortunately, we are often impatient, not trusting that if we pause and use our tools, just the right state of mind and body, just the right rhythm, will emerge without effort or manipulation. Instead, we often inhibit this process by allowing our minds to either dredge up the past or imagine scenarios that haven't yet happened.

At work it can be especially difficult to stay present and go with our own rhythm because of the expectations of the people running the show. They may believe that speed equals productivity. If we do not appear busy, we are presumably not being efficient. But despite the way others judge us and despite what we might think, the rhythm that emerges from presence is our most productive, most creative, and most sustainable pace.

There are times, of course, when we have to move more quickly — or more slowly — than we would like. Regardless, a more peaceful rhythm can emerge within our faster (or slower) movements when we stay anchored in using the tools. Although we may physically be moving at a pace foreign to us, internally our body/mind can be calm and aligned with the path of least resistance. This will be our most graceful rhythm for the situation at hand, where everything feels best — our sweet spot.

❧

Pick any situation in your life that has you moving far more quickly than you prefer. You are way too busy and the number of things you have to do far outweighs the time you have to do them in. Do you have a picture? You feel run off your feet. Your level of anxiety rises like floodwater. Your chest feels constricted; your breathing comes in short gasps. Your face turns red, and your hands start to shake.

At this point your unconscious throws out a thought into your conscious awareness such as *Oh my gosh, I'm losing it! What am I going to do? Presence! Let me take a moment and find presence.* You make a conscious decision to pause. Automatically you breathe into your umbrella, feel the weight of your tailbone (which acts as an anchor to the earth), and ask, *What could be easier?* You wait with Beginner's Mind, trusting that the answer that comes will be perfect for this situation. Suddenly, your movement is smoother, your chest has opened, your hands are steady. You feel better, more comfortable. You notice that each movement you make is easier, more efficient, more effective. And you ask yourself, *Is this my personal rhythm?*

It is!

Rhythm, Presence, and Our Sweet Spot

When we find our rhythm, we find it accompanies a certain feeling state. Remember this state! Recall it often. It is our sweet spot, and it can become a touchstone, a way to anchor back into presence. We start to notice that when we are outside this rhythm we are generally not in presence; we feel uncomfortable, as if we are in our bodies sideways. Perhaps we are getting a headache, or perhaps we're feeling prematurely tired, or stressed, anxious, or overwhelmed. All such states indicate that we have slipped outside of our personal rhythm, away from presence.

Regardless of the situation, our main priority is to anchor inward to the hub of our wheel — the most productive and empowered place to be. It is our center, where we are the observer, where we have greatest perspective, where rhythm emerges effortlessly.

Rhythm and presence go hand in hand; the more we are in one, the more we are in the other. When we slip out of our personal rhythm, the resulting friction can be a trigger that reminds us to pause a moment, breathe into the umbrella, feel the weight, and anchor back into our sweet spots. In this way, when we stay mindful our rhythm becomes a tool that assists us in staying in the here and now, thereby strengthening our communication network with Spirit and the Unified Field — another positive, self-sustaining feedback loop.

Getting to know our personal rhythm is getting to know the pace of our authentic selves, which isn't necessarily how we expected to live our lives. Sometimes our preconceived ideas about our pace has been skewed by past conditioning and erroneous beliefs. By staying in presence and allowing our rhythm to emerge, we get to observe our authentic nature and discover what *actually* works best for us, showing us how our lives can flow forth with ease and grace. As we become familiar with the rhythm of our authentic nature, we can use this knowledge to make conscious decisions that change our relationships and our life situations accordingly.

❧

One of the difficulties my second husband and I had during our relationship was that he moved, thought, and processed the world far more quickly than I. I often felt as if I were being dragged by the hair, gulping for air, as I was whooshed through life. Tension was my constant companion. By the end of the marriage, I believed my strength and speed to be inadequate. No matter what task I performed, I never seemed to get it done fast enough or thoroughly enough. As a result I lost confidence in my abilities.

After we separated, I no longer had to ramp up to my husband's pace; nevertheless, I felt as if I were walking on uneven ground that shifted and heaved when I least expected it. In my disempowered state I thought I no longer knew how to be. Out of desperation I began to use the tools. Over time I observed that my thought processes automatically slowed. So did my physical movements and what I was attracted to. I switched from rock to jazz, from action thrillers to romantic comedies. From being a woman on a mission to a woman spellbound by the infinite wonders around her: the audacious autumn colors of Hazeldean woods, the spectacular thunderstorms rolling through the Ottawa valley, the yellowed birch leaves dropping quietly on the path to Cattail Creek, the family of deer grazing on my friend's lawn in Pennsylvania, where I wrote the first pages of this book.

Later, when my ex-husband and I sat down to go through our separation agreement, he seemed to me to be vibrating off his chair as he became exasperated by how long it took me to make a simple decision. It occurred to me then that during the time of our marriage, we had both unconsciously altered our personal rhythms to accommodate each other: He had slowed down; I had ramped up.

As I became more deeply acquainted with the rhythms of my authentic self, the choices I made evolved as well. I loosened the reins on my obsessive household cleaning schedule (though my Russian grandmother probably turned in her grave as a result). I also gave up certain high-maintenance friends and all pets. I let go (for the most part) of trying to control my adult children's lives. I reduced the pressure on myself to get things done in a hurry.

Instead, I chose to put my hands into the earth and garden more. I took extra personal time to explore my inner life through journaling and heart-to-heart talks in a spiritual circle. I chose to allow a new man into my life, one with a rhythm closer to my own. Together we moved out of the fast city and onto an island with its slower West Coast pace.

*

Does my story mean that if you are in a relationship with someone whose rhythm is radically different from your own that you should dump that person and start again? Of course not. My story is my story. In an infinitely diverse universe, answers are also infinitely diverse. What's important is to honor our personal rhythm no matter what relationship we're in, be it with our mother or brother, our lover or friend, our boss or neighbor. The best chance of success for any relationship is to stay present, living in accordance with the pace of our authentic self. At this pace we flow with the current of the Life Force, reducing all friction in our movement. This includes physical movement, such as working at a desk, whipping our butt into shape, digging bulbs into the garden, or shooting hoops at the local playground; and spiritual movement — as our consciousness stretches and grows through both difficult and glorious life experiences.

When we respect our authentic rhythm, there is minimal wear and tear on our bodies and minds. Our endurance deepens. We feel younger and healthier. We operate at peak efficiency, doing less and accomplishing more. Quality and ease come to the forefront. Our stability increases along with our flexibility and adaptability. The different aspects of our nature become more integrated. We grow.

Anchoring into the Present Moment

All this wonderful stuff occurs naturally the more we anchor into the present moment. This process of anchoring is similar to meditating, but instead of sitting down in a quiet room with our eyes closed, we do it while in movement. In this way we can consciously feel the Life Force flowing through our tissue with our eyes open and our bodies not only moving but also working, playing, driving a car, or making love.

After all, this was the reason I got into Trager all those years ago! In the beginning I was able to connect with and bask in the Unified Field and enter places of utter lightness of being, but only while in meditation. I was unable to sustain the experience in the rest of my life. Now, many years later, I am able, more so than at any other time in my life, to bridge the spiritual and the physical, the absolute and the relative. But it takes ongoing practice, commitment, and intention, just as meditation does.

We use our tools in the same way meditators use a mantra while meditating: We return to them again and again, gently and without judgment. The difference is we use these tools all day, every day, and in all situations. This repetition creates a habit that permeates all areas of our lives. With this ongoing practice, we teach our consciousness (both above and below our waterline) that the more often we are in the present moment, the more we flow with the Life Force. The more we flow with the Life Force, the more our personal rhythm emerges effortlessly; the more we groove to our personal rhythm, the faster we move toward our authentic dreams, completing the circle, reinforcing the habit. Another positive feedback loop.

The address of the Life Force is in the present moment. If we want to connect to the Life Force, we have to go to where it is. To get there, we use the six tools we have learned. The tools are our vehicle — an ecofriendly vehicle at that — and by way of them, we arrive in the present moment and consciously connect our relative mind and body to our source. This completes the energetic circuit, making it self-sustaining and perpetual.

We welcome the creative intelligence of our Spirit into our being and our life. We actualize the infinite energy potential into our body and mind, expressing our being in the outer physical world, living 100 percent of the relative and 100 percent of the absolute. Now we really have it all!

INTERLUDE TWO

Whoa! That was a lot of information. If, after having been introduced to this plethora of data, you find yourself falling into feeling overwhelmed, pause.... There is no need to fight against old patterns — that only feeds them. Those patterns have banana peels as welcome mats; we inadvertently find ourselves slip-sliding over the threshold. Instead, we can allow our unconscious to work with us, directed by conscious questions such as *What does* ease *feel like? What does* lightness *feel like? How would* Spirit *have it be?*

Remember when, during my Level 1 Trager training, I wanted to place my hands just so, to move my partner's body this way and that, and — *voilà!* — have a miracle performed right before everyone's eyes? But rather than conjure up magic, I burst into tears, wailing, "I don't know how to do this. I'm never going to get it! It's hopeless!" Even as these challenging energies flowed through me, I was still capable (as we all are) of making a different choice. It took a while, but I learned to give myself permission to be a beginner. What would have happened if I hadn't allowed for an alternative point of view? No one would be reading this book, that's for certain!

All of us are beginners, even those like me who have been using these tools for years and years. So, be at ease. We are all in this together. Life's journey is infinitely complex. Give yourself permission to really not know. We will never understand it all. At no time do we have the whole picture.

Luckily, we don't have to have the whole picture. All we need to do is allow our body/mind to show up in the present moment. Our consciousness, which is an extension of our Spirit, our direct link to the Unified Field, will take care of the rest.

When we are in presence our ego-self gets out of the way, allowing our consciousness to naturally follow the path of least resistance, just as a stream finds the most effortless way to the ocean. This may not be as the crow flies, but it will be perfect for each of us — tailor-made.

So again, be at ease. What is it like to trust yourself not to know what will happen next?

❈

The last section of this book will look at the practical application of the Trager tools. Each chapter is a first-person, real-life example of an individual taking some or all of the tools I have outlined and applying them to situations and dynamics that are unique to them. Through these examples we will see the flexible nature of the Trager tools and how they apply to multiple situations and personalities.

PART THREE

PUTTING IT ALL TOGETHER

After the good earth
where the body knows itself to be real
and the mad flight
where it gives itself to the world,
we give ourselves to the rhythm of love
leaving the breath
to know its way home.

And after the first pure fall,
the last letting go, and the calm
breath where we go to rest,
we'll return again to find it
and feel again the body welcomed
the body held,
the strong arms of the world,
the water, the waking at dawn
and the thankful, almost forgotten,
curling to sleep with the dark.

The old wild place beyond all shame.

— DAVID WHYTE

CHAPTER THIRTEEN

The Story of a Waitress

I work as a waitress in a high-priced, fine-dining restaurant, and last year by using the Trager tools I increased my income by 20 percent while exerting less effort.

I had been a client of Audrey's for several years and had taken her Introduction to Trager workshop as well as her Power of Presence course — so I had already known about the tools. In fact, I used them in many areas of my life. But during a hectic rush at the restaurant I believed I had zero time or energy to focus on pausing, breathing, and feeling the weight, not to mention any of the other tools. There was just too much going on. Too much pressure. If I lost focus for a moment I feared I would lose track of all the tasks I had to juggle. Besides, my spinning mind and body at seven thirty on a Saturday night prevented even the idea of the tools from entering my thoughts. The restaurant industry, I believed, was a part of my life where it was nearly impossible to implement the tools. Little did I know that a microscopic virus would afford me little choice but to give it a go.

Near the end of August (the busiest month of the year), I caught a cold. Since it was midweek, during my days off, I hoped to get over it before my scheduled shifts. I drank plenty of fluids, tripled my vitamin C intake, took shots of echinacea, and stayed in bed. Despite my efforts, my cold worsened. So when Friday morning arrived, I was obliged to call the restaurant and inform them I couldn't make it.

Groggily I pulled my body out of bed. I opened the curtains. The sunlight stung my eyes. My whole body ached as I trudged to the living room and the telephone.

"Thank you for calling the Harbour Side Restaurant," the manager said. "May I help you?"

After I identified myself but before I could get another word out, the manager cut in. "I hope you're ready for a busy one tonight; the reservation book is jammed and the phone keeps ringing. What's up?"

"Well...um...I'm feeling a little under the weather," I said, my voice sounding as if I had spent ten years drinking bourbon and smoking unfiltered cigarettes.

"Don't tell me you're calling in sick! We're short staffed as it is. I've already called around for an extra server — there's no one. Tell me you'll be here. It will be a nightmare if we go with one less on the floor."

I sighed. What could I do? My friends, my co-workers, needed me. "Just give me the smallest section, okay?" I said.

"Done. And we'll do our best to get you out early."

As I inserted myself back between the covers of my bed, I knew there would be no getting out early. I'd be there till the end. How was I going to get through the shift? I didn't know. Even the walk to the living room took the wind out of my sails.

I imagined the night to come. My customers might see bright smiles, but behind the mask I'd be thinking, *What the hell am I doing here? I should be back in bed!*

I was going to suffer, no doubt about it. I would get a migraine. I would probably make mistakes too. Customers would complain. I would make no money.

As these ideas circled my brain, my body took a sudden downward turn. Goosebumps formed on my skin. Where a minute before I could talk, albeit huskily, now I could barely swallow. The room began to spin. Vomiting became a distinct possibility. The night to come loomed even worse. Not good!

From past experience, I knew self-pity only made an illness worse. In contrast to my lack of experience using the Trager tools in the restaurant, I *had* used the tools before when I was sick. I remembered a year earlier, when I had experienced a six-day stint with an intense migraine. At first, as I lay in the dark with my eyes covered by a damp cloth, I figured the best remedy for the pain was to get out of my body — and pronto. But the deeper the nail-in-my-head feeling went, the less I was able to escape it. And the more willing I was to practice something new. So, with pain as my motivator, I discovered that the underlying principles of the Trager Approach really do work in the real world.

As a result of this memory, in the hours before my Friday

night shift I imagined my head an empty bowl. I took a deep breath (as deep as I could, anyway) and kept my awareness on the in-and-out umbrella movement of my chest. I allowed my awareness to feel my body on the bed, the impression of its weight on the mattress. The choppy waters of my body/mind settled. A sense of equilibrium returned. My throat relaxed.

I realized I would have to keep this up the rest of the day and night. It was the only way to get through.

※

At ten minutes to five I walked into the restaurant with a steady gait, my uniform pressed and gleaming white.

"Thanks for coming in," the manager at the front desk said. "We'll try to keep your tables spaced out."

"Thanks," I said and kept walking. I didn't want to talk. I had already decided to prioritize my focus for the night. I would engage in no gossiping with co-workers. No idle conversation of any kind. No self-pitying thoughts. No concerns about making money. No worries about next week's schedule or the high-maintenance waiter in the section next to mine. Only my customers would take the focus off my conscious use of the tools.

I noticed the swing of my arms as I slowly walked toward the dining room. I felt my feet step down the three stairs and into my section. I paid attention to the weight of the cutlery and the wine glasses as I checked them for water spots. I noticed the friction of my rag against the window as I cleaned off a few toddler-sized handprints. I felt my lungs move in and out as if I were opening and closing an umbrella.

As the evening progressed my customers didn't seem to notice that my voice was an octave lower than normal, or that my eyes were bloodshot, or that I moved at a deliberate and unhurried pace.

Until that night I'd never realized how many moments I had to Hook-Up. I had always assumed there was no time. But I found plenty of moments: the forty times I washed my hands, the fifteen steps from the kitchen to the bar, the five seconds the bartender took to garnish my drinks, the twenty steps to the side stand, the ten seconds to lift a coffee cup out of the drawer and fill it, the dozen steps to the table. All these moments, and many more, were opportunities to Hook-Up. So when I arrived at a table of patrons, I also arrived in the present moment. I wasn't thinking of my cold, or of the things I still had to do, or of the chef having a tirade in the kitchen. Instead I looked at the person before me with fresh eyes.

Then, as the first round of customers left to be filled by a second seating, I fell behind. All of a sudden, I had to greet a new four-top at table 13 and a deuce at 12; there were three coffees and dessert cutlery to be delivered to 23; martinis were at the bar for table 22; dirty plates lay ready to be bussed at 11; and steak knives needed to be put down at 24 before the medium-rare filet mignons arrived — which could be any moment! I looked around. There was no one to help. Everyone else was in the weeds too. A thought crept into my head: *I'm losing it.* I put down the coffee I was pouring for table 23, afraid I'd spill it on my white apron — my hands were shaking that much. *I'm losing it.* The thought strummed through my brain. A chill went up my body. The room began to spin. *I'm losing it.* I wavered. Blood rushed to my head. This thought had severed my Hook-Up connection, allowing all my cold symptoms to swell up.

I placed my hands on the side stand and took a breath to steady myself. I was astonished by how a single thought — *I'm losing it* — could alter my body chemistry so radically. But there was no time to waste with personal revelations, not with a section full of people paying top dollar for superb food and service. I had to refocus. I took another steadying breath. I emptied the bowl of my mind — just for a moment. The room slowed. I wiggled my toes inside my sensible black shoes. I moved from side to side to feel the weight of my body. I asked, *What does connection feel like?* Then I put one foot in front of the other as I proceeded toward table 23 with three steaming coffees perched in my hands.

❖

By the end of the night I was amazed I had made it through my shift. But *more* amazing was all the money I had made. Not only could I feel the difference of being Hooked-Up, so could my customers. They practically threw money at me: 15 percent, 20 percent, 25 percent, another 25 percent! I couldn't believe it.

I didn't do anything differently; I was being different. And this helped me connect with my guests in an unanticipated way. My customers seemed put at ease by my state of mind and body. They had a good time and rewarded me with a couple of extra bills out of their pockets.

The rest of the weekend brought more of the same. Still

sick as a dog, I had to practice, practice, practice the tools to get through. And every shift, to my continued astonishment, was just like Friday night. Instead of grossing an average of 13 to 14 percent the way I traditionally did, I made 17 to 20 percent. And after my 3 percent tip-out to the kitchen, my 1 percent tip-out to the bar, and 2 percent to the bussing staff, that meant I netted 11 to 14 percent of total sales. Do the math: That's a 25 percent increase! Pretty impressive for someone who didn't think she could get through the first night.

So I figured, *I'll give this a shot every shift and see what happens. Can't hurt.*

❈

The next weekend I kept pausing, umbrella breathing, and feeling the weight of my body during my shifts, whether I was busy or not. My customers seemed warmer, friendlier, more congenial. All because I was Hooked-Up to the moment. And — lo and behold — I continued to make more money, while using less energy than before and having a better time in the process.

Almost every time I opened a billfold I was surprised. But I didn't want to jump the gun. I didn't want to say it was a trend. It could have been just random luck, a slew of generous customers. So before telling anyone what I was doing, I waited. And counted. Ten out of ten shifts. Nineteen out of twenty shifts. I began to feel confident that this was no lucky fluke. People actually related to me differently because I was grounded into the moment.

Again, I didn't *do* anything differently. I had been a proficient waitress for several decades and rarely made mistakes. The only difference was my state of mind and body.

With these results adding up, I told a few of my co-workers what I was doing. Without exception they had slightly blank looks on their faces, as if they didn't entirely believe me. "We all have runs of good luck," they said.

"Twenty-four out of twenty-five shifts of good luck!" I said.

"Really?"

"Yeah, *really*."

So I kept my co-workers abreast: twenty-seven out of twenty-eight shifts. Thirty out of thirty-one.

On my thirty-ninth shift, for whatever reason, a customer left me only 5 percent, which meant, after my tip-out, that I was out of pocket 1 percent — it cost *me* money to serve that customer! I tried to let it go, to look forward to the next table, but then those customers tipped poorly too. I began to worry what others might think regarding my failure.

"How's the night going?" someone asked.

For the first time in a long time I couldn't answer "Fantastic."

The whole weekend brought more of the same. It was an exercise in frustration. Rather than allowing Hook-Up to enter me, I tried. I put in as much effort as I could muster in my attempts to Hook-Up. I was determined to connect with my customers, to feel my feet, to pay attention to my breath — which to my dismay didn't work. My income dropped over 35 percent.

Midweek, during my regular days off, I pondered my situation and realized I had slowly become more interested in the outcome than in the process. It had become about the money rather than the feeling. Without realizing it, I had created more expectations around my ability to make a higher percentage, expectations that severed my connection. During my weekend of sickness, when I first started using the tools in the restaurant, it wasn't about what I'd get. It wasn't about my expectation of money or what others thought of me. It was about the feelings I received — feelings of lightness, of playfulness — even though I was sick.

Then I recalled the fifth tool: trusting yourself not to know. I remembered I was not in control of the outcome. To control the outcome was not my job. My job, my sole job, was to Hook-Up. That was it. Nothing more.

The next weekend while driving to the restaurant, I noticed the weight of my butt on the car seat, the in-and-out umbrella of my breathing. Then I asked, *What does it feel like to be without expectation?* I allowed innocence to wash over me. My expectations flew away like helium balloons released on a windy day. It happened without my applying effort. I was now ready to step into the frantic, hectic pace of the hospitality industry.

Minutes later, I parked my car, and without worrying whether I would make money or not I walked into my section, clear of expectations. Effortlessly my income rose once again.

CHAPTER FOURTEEN

The MS Story

A WOMAN WITH
MULTIPLE SCLEROSIS

I am a woman with multiple sclerosis, a neuromuscular condition that affects the sensorimotor pathways. Although I
was diagnosed fourteen years ago, I still lead an active life,
walking with only the slightest support from a cane. To give
context to my health, the people in my support group who
were diagnosed at the same time as I was are now either in
wheelchairs or dead. That being said, some people have re-
versed MS — there is documentation showing this. The dis-
ease is unpredictable; it is different in everyone I've met.

My relatively good health is due, at least in part, to the
fact that I am a proactive person. I do many things to help
myself: I have been getting semiregular Trager sessions for
about five years, I take supplements and do at least a few
yoga stretches each day, and I am a vegetarian who eats fresh
organic food.

Despite my good habits, however, I continue to be challenged. Sometimes when I get up after sitting or lying down

for a while, my legs turn spastic. And on the odd occasion I am challenged much further, when my ability to move shuts down almost totally, leaving me immobilized, unable to move or get help. This shutdown has happened to me three times.

The first time it happened, before I knew about the Trager Approach, I completely collapsed. I passed out on the floor and remained unconscious for hours. When I came to, I found myself paralyzed except for my head. The phone was four feet away and I couldn't get to it! The best I could do was think, *Well, this is how it is.* And so I just lay there and waited it out.

The second time it happened, I was sitting in a chair. My reaction was similar. Eventually, I managed to relax and slide to the floor. Once I was safely horizontal, I didn't try to go anywhere. Still not knowing Trager, I just waited it out.

Then I was introduced to Trager. Immediately, I added some of the Trager tools into my morning routine. Now, the moment I get out of bed I pause and breathe. After that I find my balance: First, I bring my awareness to the bottoms of my feet by sending golden roots into the earth and opening the valves in my arches. Next, I feel the weight of my tailbone by anchoring my imaginary tail. Only once I feel balanced do I move.

However, for years I just used the tools first thing in the morning and seldom remembered them at other times. Recently — for about six months, maybe a little longer — I have incorporated the tools into the rest of my life. A recent Power of Presence course reminded me to be mindful of using the tools more often: for example, when I've been sitting or lying down for a prolonged period, or when I have to get up in the middle of the night, or when I'm feeling drained because I've been doing too much. With practice I am able to use the tools upon remembering, which is almost all the time now; it has become a habit.

Then, just last month, the evening after my latest Trager session, my body shut down for the third time.

I woke up needing to visit the bathroom. As usual I paused and tailed, but I still felt a bit unsteady. Nevertheless I swished my tail into the bathroom and sat down on the toilet. Within seconds I noticed my legs go numb. I could not even sense my feet on the floor. Then the feeling in my arms went too. To add insult to injury, while as I was sitting helplessly on the toilet, sweat began to pour off my face — *drip, drip, drip, drip, drip....* Unbelievable! As in the previous shutdowns, I couldn't move my arms, even to reach the towel right beside me. But I could tell something else was going on — this was much worse than the last two incidents.

Now my usual pattern is that I initially freak out (*Am I going to die like this?* was my first thought). Then, fairly soon after, I turn things around and find some way to deal with the situation. This time what came to mind were the Trager tools. I paused and breathed, then asked, *What would it be like to feel the floor under my feet?* Though I didn't feel the floor right away, some of my strength and mobility instantly returned in my arms, enabling me to reach for a towel and wipe my face.

Next I asked, *What would it be like if my legs were more flexible?* I waited for an answer. I checked in with my knees. I could feel them! They were functioning. I relaxed and kept my awareness on the weight of my body as it slid to the floor, making sure my knees landed softly.

From the floor I asked, *What would it feel like if my legs moved slowly?* A moment later I began to crawl to my bedroom. It's amazing how fast my body came back! Using my sheets for leverage, I pulled myself up with my arms. I flopped onto the mattress and passed out.

When I woke up and reflected upon my shutdown, I realized the importance of what had occurred. I was sweating! It may not seem like much to the average person, but people suffering from MS have huge issues concerning heat. Personally, I never used to sweat. My temperature gauge had been broken for decades. I wasn't able to tolerate heat, no matter if it was from a furnace or heated muscles after exercise. And when it came to summer sun, I could handle only five minutes before feeling as if I were burning up. I just couldn't stand it; I had to find shade. So you can understand how momentous it was to be sweating.

At that moment I knew deep down that it was because of Trager. I had been told that Trager could have such effects, but I had never before experienced them so dramatically. I had only been using Trager for balance, not realizing it could also affect my biochemistry.

Trager has changed my life. It has shown me that my body can work differently. I think that having this knowing gives me more confidence to live my life normally instead of looking at myself as a victim of MS.

It is now the middle of summer, and I have been in the sun for a couple of hours every day. Though I'm still sensitive to heat, I'm aware of how much more I can tolerate. My temperature gauge is working better, and best of all I can cool down because I'm sweating! Whoopee!

❧

Although I had been getting Trager treatments for five years, I've only just woken up to its possibilities. I'm amazed at how long it has taken me to catch on. I've taken several courses. I've used Mentastics exercises. But only now have I realized that, yes, I need to use the tools *all* the time. Forming the habit of using the tools *all* the time — that's the big thing.

I now know that the Trager tools can help me get through my days more comfortably. It's not as if the MS is gone, but it's certainly a lot better; it's easier to find my balance and to move around. Today I made four dishes in the kitchen, did a little vacuuming, and, when I was through, painted my nails. It has been years since I have been able to do this. I feel as if I've been allowed to become part of the world again. It's awesome.

People with MS and other debilitating dysfunctions often think there is nothing they can do — that their condition is permanent and will never change. Many of them would call me nuts if I told them they could get positive results by talking to their legs. And maybe I am nuts, but, hey, if I'm a nut I'm in better shape than most! I do think it's important to find what works best for each individual. Certainly Trager has worked for me.

Trager has helped me get to a place of confidence in my

body and comfort with it. I know I couldn't have arrived here on my own; I didn't even remember what confidence or comfort felt like. The Trager tools have introduced to me another way of being — a healthier, more balanced way. My body now knows it is capable of doing things differently. And that sense of knowing, I believe, helps me not to give up... *ever*.

CHAPTER FIFTEEN

A Novelist's Story

When Audrey asked me to write a short essay detailing the impact of the Trager tools on my creative process I said, "No problem," figuring it would be a cinch to whip up a few pages. To my surprise, when I nestled up to my keyboard I was unable to proceed, not knowing where to start in so short a piece.

I have been told I have a block against pieces of diminutive size, that I can't help but be drawn to the nuances and details (not to mention the paradoxes). And perhaps it's true, because as I stared at my blank LCD monitor, all the repercussions of the Trager Approach on my writing life threatened to sprawl into another whole book, or at least something many times longer than Audrey had requested. I had to find a single thread around which I could weave the essay. I need not meander through my entire carpet of experience; a single idea would do. But which one? I did not know.

After an hour of bashing my brain — and receiving only bogus ideas — I decided to use the very tools I was supposed to be writing about. I let my hands fall from the keyboard to my sides. I put in my skyhook. I became aware of my bottom against the chair. I inhaled with my umbrella, and breathed out my self-inflicted pressure, my mind emptying.

Once again I had been trying too hard, exerting too much effort in an attempt to wring out a few nuggets of inspiration, which is as about as effective as trout fishing while stomping in the shallows calling out, "Come here little fishy, come here!" But such has been my pattern: I make a ruckus in my mind as I cast into the river of my imagination, trying to hook into something, anything. This was my approach for nearly half a decade, and as a result I had better success burning myself out than writing good stories.

If Trager has taught me anything, though, it has taught me to ease up when I find myself against a block — trying to bash through only lends it strength. So, still sitting in front of my blank LCD screen, pausing, breathing, and feeling the weight, I innocently tossed out a couple of questions to my unconscious: *Where is the door into this essay? What could be the central thread?*

Then I waited, doing my best to be without expectations. Yes, I waited. And waited.

The answer didn't seem to come. All I wanted to do was get up and go outside. But I had promised this essay by week's end and had allocated this evening to write at least a first draft — I didn't want to be late. My old conditioning said I should keep my nose to the grindstone. Yet my mind felt like a tight spring. I paused, breathed, and shifted my weight in my chair, noticing the vertebrae in my neck. *Where is the door?* I asked, opening myself to receiving something, anything.

Still, all I wanted to do was get up and go outside.

Well, okay, I thought. *I can trust this feeling.* And so I embarked on a trek to the local grocer. (A practical guy, I figured I'd hit two birds with one stone — get some fresh air *and* pick up dinner.)

Stepping onto the sidewalk, I glanced over at my neighbor's newly renovated home and thought of how I should have been able to buy a house of my own by now. After all, I'm nearly forty. Then a glinting Harley Davidson motorcycle caught my eye. It was a rumbling low-ride fat boy. And although I'll never be a Harley man (a BMW is more to my taste), I nevertheless coveted the country rides I could have gone on if I owned one. After that a pair of pretty young girls walked past. Like the Harley, they glinted. The low sun caught the sparkles in their eye shadow and the jewels in their pierced belly buttons. I found myself wondering if my hair looked good and if my shirt was tucked in.

At the local Petro-Canada I saw a man who was obviously a weight-pumping junkie. I glanced down at the bulge in my belly. His cut physique reminded me I had yet to get in shape. Then I thought about the old friend who had sold me a dumbbell set, currently collecting dust in the basement. I had run into him only the night before, coming out of a movie. His girlfriend was with him. I knew her too, though for the life of me I couldn't recall her name. It was embarrassing. I pictured the hurt expression on her face and wished I had the kind of brain that retained such things as people's names. It wasn't as if I didn't care. I did. Which reminded me I had to phone my close buddy, Greg — it had been way too long. And while I was at it I needed to call my family. How long had it been since I'd talked to them? A month?

The next thing I knew I was under the fluorescent lights of the grocery store. So far it had not been the relaxing stroll I had wanted. I had been spinning, I realized, as I grabbed a yellow plastic basket. My thoughts had revolved only around me. I had not really seen or heard anything of the *real* world outside myself. I was looking through the goldfish bowl of my beliefs, which put me smack-dab in the middle of an egocentric point of view. This was bad news. As a writer I need to be able to get outside my point of view at will so that when I inhabit the minds of my characters I will not be distracted by who *I* think they should be and what *I* think they should do. Having a single point of view may work for some writers, but for me (a writer who prefers the omnipotent voice) it is the kiss of death.

A writer must not allow his ego to warp his vision of the world, I continued ranting to myself as I placed a couple of lamb chops in my basket. *I must be able to open my mind and receive the diversity that is everywhere if I am to have freshness and longevity in my work.* "Do you know who is smart enough to make good fiction?" I mumbled to two beefsteak tomatoes I selected to grill along with the chops. *Not me*, I answered. *All my best ideas have come from a place* beyond *me. I translate them, of course. I write them down, organize them, edit them, but I am no more responsible for creating them than a gem cutter is responsible for compressing carbon into diamond.*

As I unloaded my few groceries onto the black conveyer belt, my cashier, a good-natured middle-aged woman with round cheeks, round eyes, and short impossibly thick gray hair, said, "Good to see you again." Her name was Charlene. I had seen her many times, just as I had given myself this speech many times. I was in familiar territory.

"Good to see you, too," I said absently, realizing my perception had again turned egocentric. Instead of actually getting out of my goldfish bowl, I had been berating myself on the importance of getting out. In other words, I was talking rather than doing. I had not yet committed to releasing my thoughts and *truly* opening to the present moment. It's a fact: The hardest part is the first pause, especially for someone whose mind slips into high gear seemingly all by itself.

So when I walked out into the evening air, I physically stopped my body as a way to confirm my commitment. Standing still just to the side of the automatic doors, I inhaled into my umbrella. When my umbrella was fully expanded, a small space of silence emerged between my thoughts. I moved into this space and kept my focus there. I felt the grocery bags balanced in either hand.

A few breaths later I started walking again, but instead of returning home the way I came, I crossed the street into the Ross Bay Cemetery. I noticed my balance shift from one foot to another, from one hip to another, as my feet carried me along a path through the historic graveyard, with its angels and crypts scattered beneath a mature and varied garden of trees. Their long shadows had cooled the air, while the ocean had infused it with the salty tang of seaweed. Goosebumps puckered on my skin. Another breath found its way deep into my lungs. On the exhalation something unwound, like the spring of a watch uncoiling all at once.

I emerged out of the trees and gazed twenty-five miles

across the choppy Strait of Juan de Fuca to the jagged edges of the Olympic mountain range awash with the last glow of daylight. The lower clouds looked like dark purple cotton balls that had been torn to pieces and carelessly tossed into the wind by a clumsy celestial infant, while the clouds in the higher atmosphere were akin to the belly of a lizard, its textured hide stained smoky red. To the west, over at Clover Point, the tourist parking lot was lined with cars, the occupants of which were no doubt watching the heavenly display above them.

I headed the opposite way along the breakwater, where thin chains of surf were collapsing against the pebbled shore. Just outside the kelp beds, the tide pulled past a tiny island of matted seaweed bearing three gulls. A cormorant shot off a rock and skimmed missilelike two inches above the water, out of my sight. The bird had been disturbed by two girls who had just sat on a piece of driftwood that could have been mistaken for a telephone pole. As I approached I recognized them as the pair I had seen on my way to the grocery store. Despite the growing dimness I was close enough to observe one shudder. Then after an instant of silence — the briefest of held breaths — she erupted into tears. Her friend consoled, "My mom's a pharmacist; she can get you a pill. I hear it's like having an extra period."

Feeling like an intruder, I quickly stepped up my pace and looked to the darkening sky. The wind had strengthened, turning the ragged purple cotton balls into an eastward marching army, somber and stern.

I had first passed those girls not fifteen minutes before and had never truly seen them for who they were. I was oblivious to the anguish that must have been on their faces. All I saw was glitter. I had been preoccupied by my own concerns. *But to be a storyteller I need to keep my perception open, my senses keen. A writer must remove his blinders and see the world clearly if he is to have any chance*...

I realized my mind was moving into high gear once again.

Far enough from the girls now, I slipped out of gear, my body slowing to a stop. Once again I had to confirm my commitment to release my thoughts and stay receptive to the world both inside me and around me. Gently yet wholly my attention returned to my breath, and the pauses I found there.

Less than a block later, under the high, knuckled oak trees of Hollywood Crescent, I realized the answer to my earlier questions: *Where is the door into this essay?* and *What could be the central thread?* had been answered. My walk around the neighborhood was the answer. The progression of experiences I moved through mirrored my creative process perfectly. Without knowing it, I had taken the route of least resistance by trusting the feeling to get up and go outside.

❦

Back at my desk, I jotted down: "When I allow myself to enter wholly into the present moment, the bounty of an infinitely creative universe comes to me." And then I explained what I meant by way of a metaphor: "Being an artist is like being a fisherman," I wrote, "except instead of fishing the Pacific or Atlantic Ocean, an artist fishes the ocean of infinite possibility, what Audrey calls the Unified Field. By way of the tools, I enter the present moment, and thereby spread an invisible net out into the ocean of the Unified Field. I don't have to do anything. I don't have to be anything. All I need is to allow moments of inspiration to swim freely into the net of my awareness."

"After all," I kept scribbling, in a groove now, "over the past few years haven't I done exactly this in all my productive studio sessions? I've used the tools to enter into the present moment of my fictional world. If my past conditioning kicks in, as it did before my walk, and I start to make a ruckus in my mind, I pause and Hook-Up. (Past experience has shown me that if I don't, I rarely get anywhere; or worse, I wear myself out spinning in circles.) When I've got a feeling of openness, I wait and listen to see if there is a scene or piece of dialogue already in my imagination. If there is, I write it down. If not, I ask a question, something like *What is Gabriel Walker* [a character in my latest novel] *looking at?* — and pause with open attention for the answer. When it comes I write it down, too, and wait for something else to happen. If nothing happens, I ask another question and again wait with open attentiveness. I keep this up until a flow comes, then I scribble like a madman until it stops. When it stops, I reconnect using the tools and ask another question. Building stories is, for me, this simple. It is an ebb and flow of questions and answers, a rhythmic process of attentiveness alternated by activity.

"The six Trager tools have revolutionized my creative process. They have helped me to get in touch with *the place* from which my creativity rises, *the place* out of which all my stories manifest. Without them I'd still be a mediocre, burnt-out writer."

CHAPTER SIXTEEN

Milton's Visitation
AUDREY'S STORY

I t was a gift.

In May 1997, four months after he had passed on, Dr. Milton Trager came to me in a dream. But it wasn't just any dream. In it I felt awake, as awake as I do now typing these words. That's why I prefer to call it a visitation.

It was around five o'clock in the morning, that time when consciousness hovers just below the surface and our creative juices run rampant through our dreaming self. Dr. Trager stood right in front of me, with his white, frizzy Einstein-like hair and crooked, boyish grin. He lifted his enormous bear-paw hands before him, palms out, fingers pointing to the sky, wordlessly beckoning me to join my palms with his. Without thought or hesitation, I eagerly obeyed, trusting him completely. His hands were supple, like soft mitts.

Then he spoke. "Are you ready?"

His question was a lightning bolt through my system.

Holy shit, this is a profound moment, I thought. At once my mouth went dry. I swallowed the last trickle of saliva; it was like downing a golf ball. Armor clamped around my chest. The feel of his palms on mine started to fade.

But I want this, I affirmed to myself. *I want this connection!*

So I paused, and breathed into my umbrella, paying attention to the weight of my rib cage expanding, then contracting. In and out, in and out. The armor began to dissolve. After what seemed like eons, my small voice bravely choked, "Yes. . . . I'm ready."

With our palms still connected, Milton gently lowered his forehead onto mine, our third eyes touching, then melding. He started toning a remarkable sound I'd never heard before. To my uneducated ear it had no discernible rhythm, but the vibration elicited waves of charged energy surging up from the earth, along his body, and passing by way of his hands and forehead into me. Wave upon wave of this energy flowed through me. My every cell opened and drank, thirsty for this newfound nourishment.

❧

The next thing I remember, Dr. Trager and I were lying side by side on a mat, watching some sort of instructional movie. He placed his left hand on top of my right hand. Arcs of blue electricity danced around our joined hands. Again I felt waves of energy wash through me. I was being instructed in some sort of knowledge that in that moment I could not comprehend. It wasn't intellectual; it was a multidimensional, energetic shift. It was beyond time. It was a year; it was a second; it saturated everything: my past, present, and future; my body, mind, and Spirit.

Gently, Dr. Trager faded away. Moments later I got out of bed and kissed my hands, immediately realizing I had not been sleeping. It had not been a dream. Dr. Trager *had* come to me.

But even before breakfast my doubting intellect got in the way. *Was it merely a dream? Was I hallucinating? Am I harboring illusions of grandeur? After all, why me? I wasn't included in Milton's circle of favored practitioners, so why would he bestow this incredible experience upon me?*

Another voice from deep inside rose to answer these doubts. *What does it matter the label I put to it?* this voice said. *Without a doubt the experience was real. I am changed. The* why me? *question is irrelevant. It happened — that is all I need to know.*

❧

Later that day I had a new client booked for a Trager session. We had met a few weeks before at a party where we found ourselves chatting, and by the end of the night she had made an appointment. Throughout the morning I looked forward to showing her (and myself) how deeply my touch had been affected by Dr. Trager's visitation. Of course, I wouldn't tell her what had happened — I didn't know her well enough for that. Nevertheless my ego-self was rubbing her hands together, chortling with glee: *Just wait until these hands get to work; she's going to experience bodywork like she's never experienced it before!*

By the time my new client arrived at my door, my mind had circled the experience at least a hundred times. Quickly we reconnected. Her bubbly, easygoing personality made it easy; before I took her coat she had me laughing.

As her slight frame moved toward the treatment room, my experienced eye noticed that contrary to her outgoing demeanor, her shoulders were slightly stooped, suggesting a contracted chest.

After the interview portion of the session, I let her know that while she was on the table she had permission to express any sounds that bubbled up, whether they were laughter, shouts of anger, cries of sorrow… even gas. I also asked her to tell me if she was feeling any form of discomfort, whether physical or emotional. "Although Trager is very gentle," I said, "it goes very deep. And I want you to feel safe."

With that, I left the room so she could undress and slip under the blankets on the table. After washing my hands, I returned and knocked softly. When I heard her say, "Enter," I quietly stepped back into the room. She was lying face up, the covers pulled up to her chin. I walked around to the head of the table and mounted it just the way I would mount a horse. (My table and I are bonded the way I imagine a cowboy and his horse are bonded.)

I closed my eyes. It was time to put the brakes on all that had happened to me that day. I breathed into my umbrella, sinking my awareness down my tailbone, feeling its weight. Slowly and gently I laid my hands on her slim shoulders and waited for the feeling of Hook-Up, that feeling that tells me my client and I are connected to each other and to the Life Force. I waited and waited, and I waited, but it didn't come. Instead of the profound *ah-ha* I had anticipated, the connection seemed shallow. My hands felt numb. My awareness couldn't get past the skin and bones, never mind sinking deeply into the Unified Field — not what I expected. I expected something more, not less. *What should I do?* I thought, but I was unable to quiet my mind enough to hear an answer. So I answered myself: *I guess I'll just start by playing with some movement.* And so I began rolling her long, slender neck from side to side. My movements seemed awkward, spastic, as if I was a brand-new beginner. I became confused and disheartened, my confidence fading fast. I knew a pause was in order, so I stopped, dismounted the table, and stepped away, breathing into my umbrella in an attempt to find connection. In my mind I asked, *How could my connection go deeper?* Numbness was the only answer. I pleaded and bargained. I pledged undying devotion to Spirit, and...silence. My ego-self cried out, *Wake up in there! Why can't I feel the Life Force?*

Still...nothing.

My chest deflated. I hung my head and surrendered to the realization that I was not going to get the results I expected. Thus far, instead of being the best session ever, it was probably one of the worst — at least from my perspective.

My ever-so-patient client had continued to lie still with her eyes closed, breathing peacefully as she waited for the session to continue. I stepped to the side of the table. It was time to end this fiasco. It would be unfair to continue the session. I reached for her arm to get her attention. My hand was a mere inch away, hovering above her shoulder, when in a flash the fifth Trager tool came back to me, the fundamental tool of receiving: trusting myself not to know what was going to happen next.

I had been projecting my expectations onto the session, not allowing my unconscious the opportunity to show me something different. I figured I knew what this experience was going to be like. No wonder I didn't feel connected! I wasn't showing up in the present moment, even though my ego-self was pretending to show up.

Okay, I thought. *I'll let go of the outcome and be with how it is. How would it feel to move into the present moment with Beginner's Mind?*

I paused once more, breathed in fully, expanding the front, back, and sides of my belly and chest. Then I felt the weight of my tailbone and continued on. This time my hands explored her tissue as if they had never done this before, taking the time to really feel. *What is this under my hands?*

A great weight lifted off my shoulders as I brought my full attention to the weight of her arm. From that point on, throughout the rest of the session I asked with genuine innocence, *What could be softer here? What could be lighter there?* No longer was I projecting a specific feeling experience; I trusted that the moment was unfolding perfectly.

When the session ended, I draped my client and helped her off the table. She smiled and said, "My chest feels so open and light!"

I urged her to look in the full-length mirror I have hanging on the wall of my treatment room to visually anchor the difference in her posture. She placed her hands on her newly expansive chest and then laughed in delight at the changed person she saw in her reflection: She stood taller, more self-assured, yet softer. She turned, her cheeks rosy, her blue eyes sparkling. "Maybe I'll fly home instead of driving my car," she announced.

❧

That morning Dr. Trager gave me, by means of the "measles principle," a key, a feeling. This flow of energy opened an inner portal, introducing me to yet another dimension of the Life Force, a dimension previously outside my experience, a dimension where joyousness and lightness is a way of being. In the years since, this experience has become an anchor, something I recall time and again. As a result the characteristics of this new dimension have continued to unfold not only when I'm working, but also when I'm washing clothes, buying groceries, going for walks, touching those I love. . . .

A Few Last Words

So here we are, at this journey's end. You have read the words and practiced the Mentastics. You have learned to use the Trager tools and are beginning to recognize the importance of consistently living in the present moment.

The Trager Approach asks us to change the way we live in the world, to transform our personal paradigm. It asks us to trust in something other than our ego-self to direct our life. It asks us to let go rather than push, to stop trying and allow each moment to unfold. It asks that we look around and notice the nonlinear intelligence that is everywhere. To be without firm expectations and enter situations without putting them in a box. The Trager Approach asks that we trust our Spirit, the central thread connected to the Unified Field, to guide us on a path specifically tailored for our uniqueness.

This uniqueness, this individuality is why the six Trager tools are flexible and adaptable. They are an *approach* to living, not a code of conduct or stringent mode of behavior. We are all unique, and the way we use these tools will also be unique. Some people start with the breath and then go to a pause. Others start with a question. Still others go to their body's rhythm first. The tools are circular; one reinforces and leads into the others. Trust your inner guidance.

Likewise, the effects these tools will have on our lives will be unique. As the few personal stories have shown, the expression of the tools are as varied as we are. What is the same for all of us, though, is where these tools take us: beyond the boundaries of our conditioning to a place of lightness, of bliss, of peace.

These feelings do not override other feelings, however. We don't become "bliss ninnies" cavorting through the tall grasses exclaiming, "Isn't life wonderful!" When my stepfather died and my mother was in shock on New Year's Day, opening to the flow of the Life Force did not negate my grieving. But the quality of my grief changed.

I didn't close down because of the emotional intensity, painful though it was. I opened to it. The tools arrived like a charging cavalry come to save the day. Virtually the entire two weeks I was in my mother's home I stayed close to the hub of my wheel. My nervous system did not become overwhelmed. I was both *in* the experience and the observer of it. As a result I didn't relate to it as an assault on my system; my ego did not put up defenses. This was a seminal time for me, the first time I had consistently used the tools in *real life*.

Certainly the memory of my stepfather's death is always with me, but because I constantly redirected myself back to the present moment, the tragedy did not stick to the conduit of my body/mind. Therefore, I was able to fly back to Ontario without additional emotional baggage.

If I had not committed myself to using the tools, the stress of the experience on my nervous system would have been like chiseling a line in concrete — it would have stayed virtually forever, creating multiple holding patterns. But because, for the most part, I allowed the experience to unfold in the present moment, the stress became more like a line on sand — with a few brushes of my hand my nervous system regained its resiliency. (Of course, if *all* of me could have stayed in presence *all of the time*, the stress would have been more like a line drawn on water!)

Contrary to what some people might expect, there were many times at my mother's that were, in their way, beautiful. Employing the tools allowed the energy of the Life Force to flow into many moments: while feeling the weight of my mother's hand, during my sister's embrace, when I slipped my arm around my mother's slim waist after the memorial service, the way our family bonded together...

Whenever we allow the Life Force to flow, a sense of beauty and wonder follows. We don't need the intensity of tragedy to focus our attention onto the present moment. We can do it anytime, during awkward and uncomfortable times, during sweet and uproariously funny times, even during blah and ho-hum times. Regardless of the situation, life can resonate with a magical quality if we bring our attention wholly to the present moment.

The more we make a habit of pausing, breathing into our umbrella, and feeling the weight, the more we will strengthen our conscious connection to the absolute, wiping clean the filters through which we perceive the relative world around us. In this way, we will respond to situations with empowerment rather than self-doubt.

Ask any world-class athlete which is more important — an intellectual understanding of the sport, or the ability to get in "the zone." In contests between athletes of similar skill, the ones who always win are the ones who don't get distracted by egoistic head talk about past mistakes and missed opportunities. They remember their strategies, of course, but they also let them go. They stay utterly committed to the present moment. The pressure of a crucial point becomes a trigger that deepens that commitment. Within the confines of their sport, they have over the years worn a groove along which the feeling of presence effortlessly flows through their body/mind.

The challenge is the same for us — conditioning ourselves to live in the present moment. Once we have the intellectual understanding, we can let it go. There's no need to overanalyze. If we focus too much on the intellectual, we miss the experience. We want the energy of the Life Force to flow, unimpeded by past beliefs and holding patterns. And, like athletes in training, we need to practice this. But unlike athletes, we don't have to reserve hours a day for it. Instead, we use the tools alongside everything we do. We pause and get into the moment, the feeling.

If, however, we find that at times we're not using the tools, there is no need to get upset or berate ourselves. Instead, as in meditation, we bring our attention back to the tools — without hoopla, fanfare, or drama. We are committed, but we are also forgiving. We're all beginners here.

Walking this path is worthy of celebration. Trust in your

own process, in the path of least resistance your Spirit has laid before you. In every moment say yes to the feelings that come from the unfettered flow of the Life Force. Allow the power of presence a permanent home in your awareness. Join me on a journey into healing — into the light.

Not until we experience it,
Is it more than just words

After we experience it,
There is no need for words.

The value of words
Is to stimulate the
Desire to experience.[7]

— MILTON TRAGER

ACKNOWLEDGMENTS

A heartfelt thank you to the following people. Without them, I would never have finished this project.

To Kyla Roodman, for planting the seed to write a book in the first place. To Candis Graham, for nurturing the tender shoot. Her gentle teaching when I was a fledgling writer and later her kind encouragement as she edited my pages were instrumental in coaxing this book to life. I will always remember her saying to me, "Give me more; I want to know more." To Susan Healey, for helping the seedling to grow strong. She provided valuable feedback on my early pages and taught me the basics of writing a proposal. To Deane Juhan and Jessica Turken, who suggested I prune my ideas to a single theme. And to those who contributed their stories — you know who you are. Your experiences and your belief in Dr. Trager's work are a source of inspiration.

To my publisher, Linda Kramer, for believing in my manuscript and giving me all the time I needed. To Managing

Editor Kristen Cashman and Editorial Director Georgia Hughes at New World Library, and to freelance editor Nancy Grimley Carleton, who was the book's final editor. It was a dream come true to find such a professional, talented, and supportive team.

And finally to Paul Latour, my partner, my love. He had the patience and courage to sit with me day after day, pruning shears and shovel in hand, as we crafted this book. His unwavering faith was a steadying force as I traversed the many rocky patches of my journey.

ENDNOTES

Book epigraph: Milton Trager, unpublished class teachings, 1975–1997.

Part 1: The Basics
Epigraph: Milton Trager, unpublished class teachings, 1975–1997.

Chapter 1: So, What *Is* Trager Anyway?
1. Milton Trager, unpublished class teachings, San Diego, 1979.

Chapter 5: Clear Communication
2. Milton Trager, unpublished class teachings, 1975–1997.

Chapter 6: But What If I Can't Feel?
Epigraph: Paul Latour, unpublished poem, 1997.

Part 2: Tools to Get There
Epigraph: Robert Bly (trans.), *Kabir: Ecstatic Poems* (Boston: Beacon, 2004), no. 14.

Chapter 9: Pause . . . Breathe . . . Feel the Weight
Epigraph: Susan Healey, unpublished poem, circa 1987.

Chapter 10: Questioning

3. Foundation for Inner Peace, *A Course in Miracles*, Vol. II (Workbook for Students) (Farmingdale, NY: Coleman Graphics, 1975), lesson 1.
4. Foundation for Inner Peace, *A Course in Miracles*, Vol. II (Workbook for Students) (Farmingdale, NY: Coleman Graphics, 1975), lesson 7.

Chapter 11: Trusting Ourselves Not to Know

Epigraph: Foundation for Inner Peace, *A Course in Miracles*, Vol. I (The Text) (Farmingdale, NY: Coleman Graphics, 1975), chapter 14; Foundation for Inner Peace, *A Course in Miracles*, Vol. II (Workbook for Students) (Farmingdale, NY: Coleman Graphics, 1975), lessons 361–65.

5. Quoted in Jack Forem, *Transcendental Meditation, Maharishi Mahesh Yogi and the Science of Creative Intelligence* (Toronto: Clarke, Irwin, 1973), p. 102.

Chapter 12: Finding Our Rhythm

6. Milton Trager, in Jack Liskin, *Moving Medicine: The Life and Work of Milton Trager, M.D.* (Barrytown, NY: Station Hill, 1996), p. 33.

Part 3: Putting It All Together

Epigraph: David Whyte, *Fire in the Earth* (Langley, WA: Many Rivers, 1999), p. 55.

A Few Last Words

7. Milton Trager, unpublished class teachings, 1975–1997.

BIBLIOGRAPHY

Bly, Robert, trans. *Kabir: Ecstatic Poems*. Boston: Beacon, 2004.

Braden, Gregg. *Walking between the Worlds: The Science of Compassion*. Bellevue, WA: Radio Bookstore, 1997.

Chopra, Deepak. *The Way of the Wizard: Twenty Spiritual Lessons for Creating the Life You Want*. New York: Harmony/Crown, 1995.

Choquette, Sonia. *Your Heart's Desire: Instructions for Creating the Life You Really Want*. New York: Three Rivers/Crown, 1997.

Denniston, Denise, and Peter McWilliams. *The TM Book: How to Enjoy the Rest of Your Life*. Allen Park, MI: Versemonger, 1975.

Forem, Jack. *Transcendental Meditation*. Toronto, ON: Clarke, Irwin, 1973.

Foundation for Inner Peace. *A Course in Miracles*, Vol. I (The Text). Farmingdale, NY: Coleman Graphics, 1975.

———. *A Course in Miracles*, Vol. II (Workbook for Students). Farmingdale, NY: Coleman Graphics, 1975.

Juhan, Deane. *Job's Body: A Handbook for Bodywork*. Barrytown, NY: Station Hill, 1987.

———. *Touched by the Goddess: The Physical, Psychological, and Spiritual Powers of Bodywork*. Barrytown, NY: Station Hill, 2002.

Liskin, Jack. *Moving Medicine: The Life and Work of Milton Trager, M.D.* Barrytown, NY: Station Hill, 1996.

Maharishi Mahesh Yogi. *Science of Being and Art of Living*. New York: Penguin/Meridian, 1995.

Marciniak, Barbara J. *The Pleiadian Times* (Raleigh, NC: Bold Connections), no. 9 (Mar. 20, 1995).

Myss, Caroline. *Anatomy of the Spirit: The Seven Stages of Power and Healing*. New York: Harmony/Crown, 1996.

Redfield, James. *The Celestine Vision: Living the New Spiritual Awareness*. New York: Warner, 1997.

Tolle, Eckhart. *The Power of Now: A Guide to Spiritual Enlightenment*. Novato, CA: New World Library, 1999.

Trager, Milton, and Cathy Hammond. *Movement as a Way to Agelessness: A Guide to Trager Mentastics*. Barrytown, NY: Station Hill, 1987.

Truch, Stephen. *The TM Technique and the Art of Learning*. Toronto, ON: Lester and Orpen, 1977.

Walsh, Neale Donald. *Conversations with God: An Uncommon Dialogue*, Book 1. Charlottesville, VA: Hampton Roads, 1995.

———. *Conversations with God: An Uncommon Dialogue*, Book 2. Charlottesville, VA: Hampton Roads, 1997.

———. *Conversations with God: An Uncommon Dialogue*, Book 3. New York: G. P. Putnam's Sons, 1998.

———. *Friendship with God: An Uncommon Dialogue*. New York: G. P. Putnam's Sons, 1999.

Whyte, David. *Fire in the Earth*. Langley, WA: Many Rivers, 1999.

Wolinsky, Stephen. *Quantum Consciousness: The Guide to Experiencing Quantum Psychology*. Norfolk, CT: Bramble, 1993.

INDEX

L

M

See also holding patterns, re-
    leasing
procrastination, 96, 98–99, 100
productivity, 158
protective mechanisms, 69, 71–72
protons, 19

Q

questioning, 92, 115–30, 165
    addictions conquered
        through, 123–28, 129
    answers, ways of receiving,
        123
    with Beginner's Mind,
        116–23, 129–30
    distancing from dysfunction
        during, 123
    and how the unconscious
        communicates, 115–16, 122
    power of, 118–19
    recall/memory in, 118–19
    revelations through, 128–29
    during Trager sessions, 121–22
    types of questions, 116–18

R

Raffi, xxviii–xxix, xxx
receptivity, 118, 149–50
    See also finding our rhythm;
        trusting ourselves not to
        know
relative vs. absolute aspects of the
    universe, 18–20, 25, 112
resistance, 74, 75–77, 95–96
responsibilities, 39
restaurant industry, Trager Ap-
    proach applied in, 169–77
rhythm. *See* finding our rhythm
Robbins, Tom, xiv

S

self. *See* ego; identity
self-delusion, 69
self-development/healing, poten-
    tials for, xiv–xv
selfishness, 53–54
sexual abuse, memories of, 71, 79
shoulders, stiffness in, 68–69, 82
skyhooks, imagining, 78, 142
smoking, quitting, 124–28, 129
Spirit, 26, 29
    See also communication with
        Spirit
stomach problems, 68–69, 116
stress, 68–69, 159, 203
survival mechanisms, 69, 71–72
sweet spot, 150–51, 158, 159

T

TA. *See* Trager Approach
table work in Trager sessions,
    74–75
tail, sitting on one's, 78, 142
Ten Commandments, xiv
tiredness, 47, 159
tissue, softening of. *See* Trager
    Approach, Trager sessions
TM (Transcendental Meditation),
    18, 21–22
Trager, Milton, xv, xxx
    background of, 4–5
    on experience and words, 1,
        62, 205
    on Hook-Up, 3–4
    on Mentastics, 7
    on rhythm, 150
    on technique, 3, 4
    visitation to Audrey, 193–99

ABOUT THE AUTHOR

Audrey Mairi is a Trager practitioner, tutor, and teacher and a Reiki Master. She regularly holds workshops for students and therapists dealing with the connection of body, mind, and spirit.

In 1969, she began the study of Transcendental Meditation (in Canada, and later in Vittel, France) and became an associate teacher in 1976. The exploration of the mind/body/spirit connection led her to certification as a Trager Psychophysical Integration practitioner in 1985, and as a Trager tutor in 1993. She served as Canada's representative on the Trager Tutor Committee and as a member of the board of directors of Trager International.

As a spiritual seeker Audrey has traveled through Europe, North Africa, and the United States, studying the intricate interweaving of body, mind, and spirit. Her interest in energy medicine led her to become a Reiki Master and explore shamanic light body exercises, shamanic drumming, soul recovery, and holotropic breathwork.

Audrey lives — and sings with the Gettin' Higher Choir — in beautiful Victoria, British Columbia.

To book or attend a workshop by Audrey Mairi, visit www.audreymairi.com. For more information on the Trager Approach, visit www.trager.com.

H J Kramer and New World Library are dedicated to
publishing books and audio products
that inspire and challenge us to improve
the quality of our lives and our world.

Our products are available
in bookstores everywhere.
For our catalog, please contact:

New World Library
14 Pamaron Way
Novato, California 94949

Phone: (415) 884-2100 or (800) 972-6657
Catalog requests: Ext. 50
Orders: Ext. 52
Fax: (415) 884-2199

E-mail: escort@newworldlibrary.com
Website: www.newworldlibrary.com